10791543

Mystery of the Cure

The Intermittent Fasting Revelation

*How Science and the Bible Have Uncovered
the Mystery of Good Health and Weight Loss*

RONALD J. COVINGTON

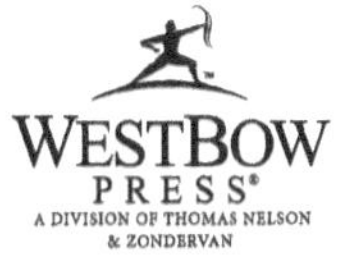

WESTBOW
PRESS®
A DIVISION OF THOMAS NELSON
& ZONDERVAN

WestBow Press books may be ordered through booksellers or by contacting:

WestBow Press
A Division of Thomas Nelson & Zondervan
1663 Liberty Drive
Bloomington, IN 47403
www.westbowpress.com
844-714-3454

ISBN: 978-1-6642-9392-2 (sc)
ISBN: 978-1-6642-9393-9 (hc)
ISBN: 978-1-6642-9394-6 (e)

Library of Congress Control Number: 2023904073

Print information available on the last page.

WestBow Press rev. date: 03/27/2023

This book is dedicated to the
memory of my best buddy of thirty-five years.
Peter Searle
1958–2020
I truly believe that if he and I had discovered and applied the
Mystery of the Cure five years ago, he would be with us today.

This book is also dedicated to the millions of faithful Christian men
and women across the globe struggling with optimizing their health as
evidenced by weight gain, as they see their bodies expand little by little
adding a pound here or there over the years. I know I did. But not anymore!
This simple little book will demonstrate how *God created* the human
body to be healthy, vibrant, and alert. By following the eating patterns as
revealed in the Bible and supported by science, you too will be energized
to live out the purpose and calling for which *He created you* to live.

One of the most discouraging things I encountered during *the first 11 years of my practice* was the fact that a very large *treatment* could be done without any vital knowledge of the *treatment* to be performed, a fact, as I told you, I got a hint of *while working* behind the *pharmacy counter.* This is really an anomaly *found only in the field of medicine.* That an intelligent, thinking, reflecting, human being will put his own life or the life of his wife or child into the hands of those who, in every scientific sense, are not well fitted to perform some of the most complicated of scientific *treatments* there are without previous knowledge or experience allowing them to *prescribe unproven medication on* the sick, is a marvel in human affairs.

As I have intimated before, this arises from the people's superstitious faith in the power of *medicine* over disease, and this faith of course arises from ignorance.

Cheer of mind is such a prime necessity to health; and *the prospect of disease,* is so gloomy a subject to even think about; that the mind recoils from thought upon it; hence results the prevailing ignorance, even in the more cultured classes, and hence the ease with which all classes alike become the prey of the spoiler in times of the emotional tension when reason has become impaired, and strong words, and strong assurances are received as cold water by a thirsty soul, even with child-like faith, no matter how founded upon ignorance. This must ever be so until the people become aware that disease is largely a condition arising from avoidable causes, and that the cure is largely a matter of *God's* own handiwork.

—Edward Hooker Dewey, MD, 1902

Contents

It was December 3, 2012, when my wife, Grace, and I were on an early season ski weekend in the Rocky Mountains of Colorado, and the conditions were less than optimal. As a matter of fact, they were horrible! The air was wet and heavy, the visibility was poor, and the temperature was bone-chilling cold. But, hey, it's Colorado! Don't be a fair-weather skier. We had been doing this for years, and the skiing was usually great even in the toughest conditions. Today of all days, Copper Mountain's state-of-the-art, world class snowmaking machines would provide plenty of fresh, Colorado Champagne powder—or so we thought. I was on my brand new, freshly tuned Volkl Tiger Sharks, and I had convinced myself that I needed to try them out since I was soon having a rematch with our friend, Peter Siegel. At the end of the previous ski season, Peter had beaten me on a short slalom racecourse, rather easily I might add, at the bottom of Brennan's Grin near the Excelerator lift.

I was eager to test my new skis on the American Flyer and show Peter he had nothing on me. The American Flyer was an intermediate blue groomer on which my wife and I had skied numerous times. There was a nice little burger shack providentially located at the bottom of the run, next to a very rustic men's and women's restroom.

Grace and I started our run sliding past a tiny little restaurant named Flyer's Grill, which our friend George affectionately called "The Fly Shack." We quickly approached a service road that was carved through the run. It was covered with snow, which enabled us to use it as a "roller," where we would roll over and catch a little air. We quickened our pace as we whisked by the snow cannons, spraying snow from the blower heads perched high upon their stainless-steel poles. Making artificial snow is a pretty common occurrence in Colorado during the early ski season due to the lack of precipitation.

We quickly came upon the oft enjoyed "roller," which, I failed to realize, had accumulated too much of the man-made snow, creating a frozen little jump located on the downhill side of the service road. The unexpected jump launched me forward, where I landed headfirst on a patch of ice in the middle of the run. There I was, lying face down, motionless, as Grace skied up beside me. She immediately rolled me face-up and, with the help of some other skiers, spun my body around so that my head was on the high side of the mountain. She then called her friend, knowing that her friend's husband was a member of the Copper Mountain patrol and rescue team.

Within minutes ski patrol arrived and quickly removed the cracked ski helmet from my head, cut the jacket off my body to avoid any further damage, gently placed me in the rescue sled, and slid me down the mountain. The patrol team took me to a local hospital in Frisco, Colorado, where they induced me into a coma and placed my limp body in an ambulance sending me seventy-five miles to an acute-care hospital located on the Front Range of the Rockies. Once there, I would lay in that state fourteen days.

Rather than being life-flighted in a helicopter, the trip to St. Anthony's Hospital in Lakewood, Colorado, took a full hour and twenty minutes because the helicopters had been grounded due to stormy conditions. The clock was ticking, and the medical staff was on alert. Doctors worked feverishly as Grace watched and prayed. After they brought me into the emergency room, doctors proceeded to insert a brain bolt through my skull to relieve the pressure and monitor brain oxygen. As it turns out, I had suffered a traumatic brain injury, with frontal lobe hematoma as well as shearing of the brain synapses resulting in my right and left frontal lobes being damaged. Before the right side of my brain could process what the left side was saying, the severed synapses would need to regenerate. The regeneration would take a minimum of eighteen months and could potentially take several years. My recovery was going to be a long one. I had to learn to eat, drink, sit up, walk, talk—everything. My brain had to do a full "reboot."

A symptom of the brain shearing was a serious lack of impulse control.

The side of my brain that would say, "Ooh, that looks really good," was no longer being tempered by the side that might counter, "Don't do it." You might say that the angel on one shoulder was being outwitted by its counterpart on my opposite shoulder with my brain having no ability to discern between the two. During my recovery and due to the sheared synapses, I became very impulsive with almost everything I did. If something made me angry, I became very angry. If I wanted to enjoy a drink, I drank way too much; if I wanted to enjoy a meal, dessert, or snack, I overindulged every time. I ate because I loved to eat—and a lot. Food was truly a comfort, I guess, but surely it was not because my body needed the energy. Was it? No. It was just a bad habit that I alone had created for myself.

Thankfully I was able to recognize this bad habit and, slowly, over the next ten years, I began to eat relatively well, but as it turns out I was eating way too often. An English muffin and poached egg in the morning sounded reasonable. Followed by a midmorning snack on some beef jerky or hummus packets to keep my metabolism hummin' along, a healthy lunch, a bag of chips in the afternoon, a relatively healthy dinner with an occasional dessert and maybe some peanut butter and crackers or peanuts before bedtime. This routine was not at all uncommon.

I weighed two hundred pounds at the time of my skiing accident. My newly adopted lack of impulse-control eating habits resulted in a modest gain of merely one-half pound per month. That's only six pounds in an entire year. All I needed to do was self-correct my impulses and reverse the trend by a mere .0164 pounds per day. I figured I could easily diet, exercise, or simply will myself to cut down my caloric intake by .0164 pounds per day, which is only a daily reduction of 57 calories. Surely, I could reduce my caloric intake by a mere 57 calories per day. Just eat a little less beef jerky or skip the occasional dessert; that should do the trick. Well, it didn't work. Ten years later, at the age of fifty-six, I found myself weighing in at 260 pounds. At my height, that is obese by any standard. I needed to improve my health and drop some weight—a lot of weight. I just didn't know how.

In January of 2022, a colleague of mine told me he was considering trying intermittent fasting because he heard some good things about it. He was skeptical as to whether he could do it because he thought it might interfere with his daily workout regimen and his weekly soccer matches. Intrigued, I began researching the topic, and like many, I did so via the internet searching for topics on intermittent fasting.

During my search, I came across an online video of Johns Hopkins University professor Mark P. Mattson, discussing the benefits of intermittent fasting. His presentation was based upon the extensive research that he had conducted during the past thirty years on the topic. His claim was that eating in time-restricted patterns had significant neurological benefits with the added side benefit of significant weight loss. I was interested in learning more, so I eagerly preordered his upcoming book, *The Intermittent Fasting Revolution,* which I received on February 1, 2022. His book contained extensive scientific evidence supporting the many health benefits of eating in the intermittent fasting pattern. The results were astonishing. Could this really be true? Increased mental acuity, more energy, and extensive health benefits accompanied by weight loss by merely changing one's eating patterns? All this without dieting, counting, measuring, or spending a lot of money on premade meals, powders, or shakes? I had to admit that it sounded too good to be true.

In his book, Dr. Mattson posits that the benefits of intermittent fasting evolved from the time-restricted eating patterns that were necessary for prehistoric humans' daily life and survival. They evolved because of millions of years of atheistic, materialist, Darwinian evolution: from abiogenesis (nonlife becoming life) to apes, to prehistoric man, to who we are today. While I can accept Mattson's findings on the numerous neurological health benefits, giving credit to an atheistic, materialistic theory of evolutionism was something I simply could not embrace.

As I was reading the Bible one morning, I happened upon the passage Exodus 16:21. For the first time, I read it with what I thought was more insight than usual. It seemed as though God was uncovering a mystery for His people in the Sinai desert on how and *when* they should eat, and He was revealing it to me that very morning thousands of years later: what time they should start, what time they should stop, and what time they were to abstain. They had to do physical work in the morning as they gathered the day's provision. Then they would prepare the manna and eat it in a window of time that would end in the early afternoon. They were to abstain from their next meal until the following morning, which would take place only after collecting that day's supply. It was as if a lightbulb went on; it was a picture of a time-restricted eating pattern, which we commonly refer to as *intermittent fasting.*

With this new discovery in mind, I began to search the Bible to see if other eating patterns in scripture might support the concept of time-restricted eating. My goal was not to make scripture conform to my new theory, nor was it to align myself with the recent fad diets that label themselves as an intermittent fasting diet plan. Rather, I wanted to see if other areas in God's Word demonstrated similar eating patterns. I came to the scriptures open-minded and started to study, and after extensive research, I found that, indeed, there were other examples of this pattern. In fact, there were many of them. The only exception I found recorded in scripture that did not follow this pattern resulted in God's judgment (see Appendix 1).

Best-selling author Eric Metaxas argues in his book *Is Atheism Dead?* that all creation resulted in a *finely tuned universe* created by God. I agree. As a matter of fact, I agree completely. Likewise, I would argue that the resulting benefits of employing the intermittent fasting patterns as demonstrated in the Bible and outlined in Mattson's book are the result of our *bodies* being created by and in the image of God. Just as He created our *finely tuned universe*, he also created our *finely tuned bodies.*

So, before we dive into the mystery of the cure, we need to address a couple of issues. First, as we shall see, the chances of us evolving for 13.8 billion years into the finely tuned human beings we are today are extremely remote. Second, according to the Bible, we were created by God in His own image in one literal seven-day period as outlined in Genesis 1:3–31. Secular science on the other hand, claims the universe is 13.8 billion years old; however, the Bible is silent on the topic. Because the Bible does not speak to the age of the universe, in this book we will be silent as well. Nevertheless, the Bible does establish the age of our earth is 6,165 years of as of the date of this publishing (Anstey 1973). Science claims life on earth has been here for 3.8 million years with mutating cells followed by 2 million years of human evolution to get us where we are today. The Bible makes it clear that God created the Earth and everything on and around it. Thus, evolution deserves no credit for our finely tuned bodies, nor will it get any from this author.

We also need to establish answers to a few simple questions before we get into the complexities of our amazing self-healing bodies. Did life emerge suddenly from some prebiotic primordial soup absent a creator as science says it did? Did this newfound life begin to split and replicate itself with the ability to evolve over billions of years into fish that grew legs, turned into dinosaurs who eventually learned to fly, then for some unknown reason migrated to graveyards where they all proceeded to die en masse and were instantly fossilized without decay, within varied weather conditions over the millennia? Did we randomly leap from nonlife to life over billions of years, evolving by chance so meticulously into the finely tuned bodies that we enjoy today? Or did God simply *speak* us into existence when He said "Let Us make man in Our image, according to Our likeness … male and female He created them" (Gen. 1:26–27 NKJV). I would put forward the latter, as we will discover throughout the remainder of this book.

Acknowledgments

Edward H. Dewey, 1837–1904

For his insights that were well ahead of their time and that challenged the medical establishment for the betterment of all.

Mark P. Mattson

For his extensive work in the field of neuroscience and uncovering the scientific benefits of intermittent fasting.

Eric Metaxas

For his work in *Is Atheism Dead?* Much of what I learned about abiogenesis and our finely tuned Earth and universe came from his work.

Pastor Dave Love

For his unwavering commitment to equipping the Saints with the knowledge and love of God's Word, as well as equipping them with the knowledge of God's love for us.

The Holy Spirit

I prayed to the Holy Spirit and asked Him to help me put these thoughts into written form if they would be of any use and bring Him glory.

Naomi Specht

For her love of the Word, attention to detail and her propensity to ask questions in her quest to seek clarity and pull out what I was trying to communicate to the reader. I couldn't have done it without her.

xvii

Introduction

> The Elder (John), To the beloved Gaius, whom I love in
> truth: Beloved, I pray that you may prosper in all things
> and be in health, just as your soul prospers.
> —3 John 1–2 (New King James Version)

In the middle of the nineteenth century in the hills of Western Pennsylvania, a Mr. Edward Hooker Dewey worked on the family farm with several of his older siblings. Young Edward, while deciding on whether to make the practice of medicine his lifework, reasoned that "there is a destiny that shapes our ends," and he was determined to find out his awaited fate. His father's farm wasn't big enough to support all his sons, so Edward decided—because of his "slight build"—he was not well suited for the heavy manual labor required of farming.

"There was a local Doctor in the area of a very wise demeanor and stately form who was in want of a medical student, and this Doctor had known a Drug Store owner who was in need of a young apprentice to learn the business" (Dewey 1894, 26–27). The young upstart, Edward, saw this as an excellent opportunity. He could simultaneously read and study medical books under the tutelage of such a well-qualified mentor, all the while learning about pharmaceuticals. In all practicality he would become a doctor right out of the gate, despite the absence of any formal medical training. He stated, "Through the door opened, I walked, never to go out again."

One of the insights that Edward discovered before he began to study medicine is "I (*he*) had become aware of the fact that the majority of persons *stricken* with acute disease recovered, no matter how (*the type of treatment), or by whom*" (ibid.). He had observed that most people, even in such rural locations using untested and unscientific remedies, had success even though they had neither the money nor the access to medical treatments. How could this be? The medical establishment was entrenched in using accepted methods for the sick that were largely unavailable to those in rural areas. Surely, they must be far less healthy than those benefitting from the established modern medical treatments and practices found within the city limits. Right? Not so.

Over time, Edward began to wonder about this mystery, and it's this mystery he would come to refer to as *the mystery of the cure.*

After receiving his medical degree from the University of Michigan, Edward found himself in charge of a military field hospital ward, which turned out to be the beginning of his professional career. The year was 1864 near the tail end of the American Civil War. Edward was stationed at a field office in Chattanooga, Tennessee, within a ward filled with cots of newly wounded soldiers fresh from the battle of Resaca, Georgia. He was unprepared for what he was about to encounter. Up to this point, he had no clinical experience. In fact, he had never had to care for a severely sick or severely wounded person and was certainly never confronted with the nearly eighty cots filled with soldiers who were "thrust" into his care. The wounds were extensive, and the number of cases were endless. Edward spent his days dressing wounds, performing the rejoining and securing of fractured bones all the while providing attentive care and comforting words of encouragement to his weary patients (ibid.).

Mr. Dewey remained on-duty treating patients for a year and a half without the clinical advantages that otherwise would have been available in hospitals. Contrary to the accepted medical practice of the time to overmedicate, Dr. Dewey's tendency was to use very little of the prescribed methods, and the medical doses of drugs that he gave to his patients were administered on a very limited scale. Drugs were used primarily to relieve pain while Nature took care of the healing process. Nevertheless, he never had any reason to believe that his services failed to reach the expected results of clinical treatments. "I must say, that I failed to have a single case where I felt certain that a human life was saved by the use of the medicines given" (Dewey 1894). The *mystery of the cure* was as deep as ever.

Over a twenty-six-year career witnessing countless recoveries from acute illnesses to observing healthy metabolic transitions, Dr. Dewey was convinced that "Divine Nature" would provide the necessary cure in most instances. The *mystery* was coming into focus.

Chapter 1

Mystery of the Word

The Angel of the LORD

In the beginning was the Word, and the Word was with God and the Word was God. [14] And the Word became flesh and dwelt among us (John 1:1, 14a NKJV).

From this passage, I want to point out and answer three common questions. Who is the Word? None other than the Lord Jesus. When did the Word begin and with whom? At the very beginning with God the Father and God the Spirit (Gen. 1:1,2). What is the Word? The entirety of scripture. It is important that we establish the mystery of the word being Jesus because it was He who led the people out of Egypt, and it was He who taught them the time-restricted eating pattern we find in Exodus 16:21.

The Gospel of John explains that Jesus did not come into existence when He was born in a barn, wrapped in swaddling cloths, and laid in a manger. No, Jesus was *with* God in the beginning, and was in fact God. The Hebrew word used for God in Genesis 1:1 is the plural word *Elohim*, which speaks of God's triune nature: Father, Son, and Spirit otherwise known as the trinity. This triune everlasting eternal creator God spoke into existence the entire universe including the Earth that we live on today.

So, the question becomes, what did the second and third persons of the trinity do after they helped create everything that was made? Did they sit back in their heavenly realm watching God the Father inspire Moses to lead the children of Israel out of Egypt, speak to Moses from a burning bush, lead them through the wilderness, and dwell with them in the temple waiting for God the Son to arrive through a virgin mother? Again, the answer is a resounding no! Scripture tells us how the Spirit inspired the prophets to pen what we now refer to as the infallible canon of scripture.

So where was the second person of the trinity, the preincarnate Christ? I would submit to you that He was actively working throughout the Old Testament from the very beginning and is referred to throughout Hebrew scripture as "the Angel of the LORD." The Hebrew word *mal'ak* is defined as a messenger, and it sometimes refers to human messengers as was the case when referencing John the baptizer in the book of Malachi where we do not find the definite article "the."

"Now the Angel of the LORD found her [Hagar] by a spring of water in the wilderness, by the spring on the way to Shur" (Gen. 16:7 NKJV).

When the definite article "the" is added to it, it always refers to Jesus (Foreman, Van Dorn 2020, 25–33). The first reference can be found in Genesis 16:7 where the Angel (mal'ak) of the LORD (Yahweh) is speaking to Hagar. In this instance LORD is referencing Yahweh, and the Angel is referring to Jesus and will do so throughout the entire Hebrew Bible.

"Then she called the name of the LORD who spoke to her, You-Are-the-God-Who-Sees; for she said, 'Have I also here seen Him who sees me?'" (Gen. 16:13 NKJV).

Here Hagar calls on Yahweh who had spoken to her and asks the rhetorical question, "Have I also here seen Him who sees me?" Yes, God the Father, God the Son, and God the Spirit make up the one true God of Israel. And because no one can see the LORD and live (Ex. 33:20; John 1:18), Hagar saw the second person of the trinity. She saw the Face of the LORD. She saw Jesus.

"The Old Testament is trying to describe how people can 'see' and 'know' God. Moses is 'seeing' the unseen God. The God of the universe, who cannot be seen, is showing [His] presence to [His] people by sending a mediated form [Who] is the presence of God. ... The glorious explanation is that this is the Son of God manifest as the Angel of the LORD in the Old Testament albeit in a deliberately mysterious way" (Foreman, Van Dorn 2020, 81).

Throughout the remainder of this book, it is important to understand that the Angel of the LORD as well as the Face and Voice of the LORD is the second person of the trinity: The Lord Jesus Christ. Jesus said so

Himself in John 14:6 when he said, "I am the way, the truth, and the life. *No one* (emphasis mine) comes to the Father except through me." This is the same Lord who *spoke* to His children throughout the Old Testament, and this is the same Lord who *speaks* to us today through His written Word: the Bible. Let's see how this very special Messenger taught His people how to eat.

Manna from Heaven

"So they gathered it every morning, every man according to his need. And when the sun became hot, it melted" (Exod. 16:21 NKJV).

Breakfast is the most important meal of the day. We have all heard this over the years, and if you haven't, then no doubt you've heard something similar. If you don't start off with a hearty protein-filled breakfast first thing in the morning, you will not have the necessary energy to make it through to lunch. In fact, some say if you start out with a protein rich breakfast, and snack continually on healthy foods up until the lunch hour, your metabolism will be humming along, burning off more energy than you take in because your body will be in a constant metabolic state—the way it is supposed to be. This is the message that's been pushed at us since we were toddlers. Even my grandma took the bait, one of the wisest women you could ever meet. "Make sure you eat something that will stick to your ribs," she used to tell me. Meaning, if you eat a good, hearty breakfast, it will set you moving on the right path so you can make it through 'til lunch.

Not so fast. While this may have been the typical way of thinking for years, is it actually true? Is this the best way to improve your metabolism, lose weight, and stay healthy? Is it possible we got it wrong when it comes to eating patterns and optimizing health? Just as the invention of the Hubble telescope in the 1940s has forever changed how scientists view the state of our universe (more on that to come), so too has modern technology changed our understanding of the benefits of adopting time-restricted eating patterns.

When considering the evidence, Dr. Edward Dewey discovered that if a person skipped the early morning meal, that person had clear and significant health benefits. He just didn't have the science to prove how it worked, nor would he have the benefit of such science throughout his medical career. As you will soon see, science now confirms that starting the day by fasting from the previous evening's meal until around lunchtime enables one's body to *optimize health and enhance performance*: both mentally and physically. The science revealed by Dr. Mark Mattson, as put forth in his book *The Intermittent Fasting Revolution*, leaves little doubt about the benefits of intermittent fasting. And as it turns out, God Himself, through Moses and Aaron, instructed the children of Israel to eat in that exact same pattern over three thousand years ago. Not only did He command it to the generation that Moses led out of Egypt, but this commandment applied to the following generation as well. In total, two generations ate in the time-restricted eating pattern of which God taught them to eat for forty years. In my mind, there is no doubt. He did this because He loved them and knew it would bless them.

The book of Exodus tells the familiar story when God used Moses to free the children of Israel from Egyptian bondage. God brought plagues upon Egypt to convince Pharaoh to free them from bondage, He parted the Red Sea, and the Angel of the Lord led them out of Egypt. The preincarnate savior of the world, Christ Jesus himself, was the one who led them into the Sinai wilderness and into the promised land. (Num. 20:16, Judges 2:1, Jude 1:5) This is where they began, with what turned out to be a very long, four-decade, pilgrimage to the land promised to Abraham and his descendants.

Two and a half months into their journey, they realized they were quickly running out of the supplies they had prepared before they escaped out of Egypt (Exod. 12:39). As a result, they started to complain mightily. The rabble rousers, as described in Numbers 11:4, got them all worked up to the point where they accused Moses and Aaron, saying that they led them out to the wilderness to die and that they were going to starve to death. The Israelite people were so distraught that they even wished they had remained slaves in Egypt where they, at the very least, would have "pots of meat" and be able to "*eat* bread to the full" (Exod. 16:3).

"Then the LORD said to Moses, 'Behold, I will rain bread from heaven for you. And the people shall go out and gather a certain quota every day, that I may test them, whether they will walk in My law or not. And it shall be on the sixth day that they shall prepare what they bring in, and it shall be twice as much as they gather daily'" (Exod. 16:4–5 NKJV).

The children of Israel cried out; God heard them, provided for them, and began instructing them on the eating pattern by which they should eat. He taught them that *when* to eat was more important than *what* to eat, and that fact stands true today. He taught them *the Mystery of the* Cure and how to *flip the metabolic switch.*

Training Camp Starts Tomorrow

Growing up, I was a huge Dodgers baseball fan. I could not wait for winter to be over, so I could watch the "boys in blue" once again make their way back to Vero Beach, Florida, to start their training camp. They needed to get into game shape, master the new signs and signals, prepare to face major league competition, and be mentally and physically fit for what would be a very long and challenging season. It was a time of intense preparation.

Similarly, Moses, Aaron, and the Israelite people were about to begin their training camp. God had a lot He wanted to teach His people before the season was going to start, not the least of which was to show them how He was going to provide for them in the middle of the Judean desert as they journeyed to the promise land. He began by outlining the pattern by which He would have them eat. He was going to give them "bread from heaven," "water from a rock," and He would provide a double portion of bread on Fridays, so they could honor Shabbat, the Sabbath day of rest. God would be the Provider of every need, and while He was teaching them, they would see the "Glory of the Lord" and "know that I am the LORD your God."

There is little doubt that back in Egypt the "pots of meat" and the "bread to the full" of Exodus 16:3 were consumed outside of God's preferred eating pattern. This act may have led to even further hostility given they were no longer able to do as such. Nevertheless, God having heard the murmuring complaints of His people and because He loved them, even though they were sinners (Romans 5:8), would grant them one last evening meal: "At twilight you shall eat meat, and in the morning you shall be filled with bread. And you shall know that I *am* the LORD your God" (Exod. 16:12 NKJV).

But no more. Twilight meals as they wandered in the wilderness were about to be eliminated. The very next morning, God's eating pattern would be given to His people. Let the training camp begin.

The Provider of Every Need

And when the layer of dew lifted, there, on the surface of the wilderness, was a small round substance, *as* fine as frost on the ground. So when the children of Israel saw *it*, they said to one another, "What is it?" For they did not know what it was. And Moses said to them, "This *is* the bread which the LORD has given you to eat. This is the thing which the LORD has commanded: 'Let every man gather it according to each one's need, one omer for each person, *according to the* number of persons; let every man take for *those* who *are* in his tent.'" Then the children of Israel did so and gathered, some more, some less. So when they measured *it* by omers, he who gathered much had nothing left over, and he who gathered little had no lack. Every man had gathered according to each one's need (Exod. 16:14–18 NKJV).

As we see here, God would not forsake the children of Israel, and it was always His full intention to provide for their every need: never to starve them. The bread that God gave them in the wilderness provided all they would need to sustain them until the following day.

The book of Numbers gives us some insight as to what this bread from heaven was like: "Now the manna *was* like coriander seed, and its color like the color of bdellium. The people went about and gathered *it*, ground *it* on millstones or beat *it* in the mortar, cooked *it* in pans, and made cakes of it; and its taste was like the taste of pastry prepared with oil. And when the dew fell on the camp in the night, the manna fell on it" (Num. 11:7–9 NKJV).

As mentioned earlier, God would provide the nutrition by way of manna (Exod. 16:21) and water by way of a rock (Exod. 17:6) to sustain them as He instructed them in the wilderness. Furthermore, He would do this for forty years. He would also teach them the pattern by which they should eat. It is the same intermittent fasting eating pattern that many have adopted today: "So they gathered it every morning, every man according to his need. And when the sun became hot, it melted" (Exod. 16:21 NKJV).

If you are anything like me, you love your early mornings. The coolness of the air, the freshness of the day, a hot cup of coffee, studying God's word. Awesome!

God also loves mornings, and why wouldn't He? He created them. We see here how God instructed His children on how to start each day. When we break it down, we find that it follows the 17–7 intermittent fasting pattern down to the "T." Each morning they would gather enough manna for each person according to his or her need. We see in verse 16 that the amount to gather was one omer per person, which is an old measuring unit of dry grains equaling about 3 liters. That meant a family of four would gather approximately 12 liters of food and have it eaten before it melted "when the sun became hot." If they were to start gathering manna around 6:00 a.m. and started eating about 8:00 a.m., they would have had a seven-hour eating window to consume the day's supply before it would subsequently melt at 3:00 p.m. Seven hours of eating and 17 of fasting: 17–7. As we will discuss later, the hottest part of each day around the globe occurs at three o'clock in the afternoon.

Additionally, in Exodus 16:21, God revealed to the children of Israel, as well as to us today, a wonderful picture of their coming Messiah. The Father provided bread from heaven daily. He also sent His Son from Heaven who was born in Bethlehem (which translates to house of bread), Who is in fact, the Bread of life. The children of Israel ate of this bdellium-colored bread. Bdellium is a gum resin similar to embalming myrrh which speaks of Christ's death. Jesus is the Word, and we are to *feast* on His Word every day. They finished eating at 3:00 p.m. when God melted the manna. Jesus, while hanging on the cross at 3:00 p.m. said, "it is finished," and committed His soul to the Father.

God was showing the children of Israel while they were still wandering in the wilderness a *type* of the Messiah to come. He was telling His story of redemption to those who would be saved by believing in the coming Savior—Jesus. God intentionally gave His son (the bread of life) at the same time of day He melted the manna to show everyone (both Jew and non-Jew) that Jesus would give His life, and that Jesus Christ is in fact,

Lord. At the very moment Jesus said, "it is finished," He went to Sheol (the place of the dead or Abraham's bosom) and set the captives free. Likely many of those captives were the children of Israel who wandered in the wilderness eager for their coming Messiah thousands of years earlier. Our God is awesome!

As we discussed earlier, God taught them this pattern for many years. It was important enough that He gave it to two generations. By doing so, their bodies would be able to optimize their overall health, and this eating method would be passed on for many generations. They may or may not have known of the benefits at the time, but, thanks to modern scientific research, we now do.

Jethro's Sacrifice and Offerings

"Then Jethro, Moses' father-in-law, took a burnt offering and *other* sacrifices *to offer* to God. And Aaron came with all the elders of Israel to eat bread with Moses' father-in-law before God" (Exod. 18:12 NKJV).

Here in Exodus we find Moses's father-in-law, Jethro, priest of Midian, taking a burnt offering to God and eating bread with Moses's brother, Aaron. This is where we can see how Jethro, a non-Jew, was following the same eating pattern that Moses taught God's people to follow in Exodus 16:21.

According to the Tamid daily sacrifice (also known as the perpetual sacrifice), Jethro's burnt offerings and sacrifices to God would have begun early in the morning. At 6:00 a.m., the first hour, the first lamb was tied to the altar and the priests prepared the altar. At 9:00 a.m., the third hour, the first lamb was to be sacrificed followed by prayer. At noon, the sixth hour, the second lamb was brought and tied to the altar and the praying continued until 1:00 p.m. At 3:00 p.m., the ninth hour, the second lamb was to be sacrificed and prayer would continue for the final hour.

The following timeline of the Tamid daily sacrifice would allow for the eating of bread spoken of in Exodus 18:12 to be consumed between the hours of one thirty and two thirty, leaving time to prepare and clean up. They would be finished eating by the "heat of the day," as commanded in Exodus 16:21. It was tradition to have the main meal in the early afternoon, and it still is to this day in the Middle East (Fruchtenbaum 2021, 283). Illustration #1

JEWISH TIME	ROMAN TIME
SCHEDULE OF THE TAMID SACRIFICE	
FIRST HOUR	**DAWN**
The first lamb is brought out and tied to the altar at dawn	The priests prepare the altar [Exodus 29:38–42; Leviticus 6:1–6
THIRD HOUR	**9 AM**
The first lamb is sacrificed at 9 AM	9 AM is the first hour of prayer [Acts 2:15] Temple gates open *Shacharit* (morning)
SIXTH HOUR	**NOON**
The second lamb is brought out and tied to the altar at noon.	Noon is the second hour of prayer [Acts 3:1, 10:9]
NINTH HOUR	**3 PM**
The second lamb is sacrificed at 3 PM	3 PM is the third hour of prayer; also called the hour of confession [Acts 3:1; 10:9]

While Exodus 18 does not record the timing of the events that we find here in the Tamid of daily sacrifices, we understand scripture makes it clear that the Jewish leadership of the day followed the oral law as it was handed down from generation to generation. We can confidently conclude that the creation of the schedule of the sacrificial system was handed down by the forefathers.

We find in Jethro's account, that the time available for them to have their main meal of the day would be between the sixth hour and the ninth hour or from noon to 3:00 p.m. Let's look at the details of this system in light of a time-restricted eating pattern.

- Dawn: The first lamb is tied up, and the priests prepare the altar.
- 9:00 a.m.: The first lamb is sacrificed, and the first hour of prayer begins.
- 11:00 a.m.: Nothing is scheduled. Potential mealtime.
- Noon: The second lamb is tied up, and the second hour of prayer begins.

- 2:00 p.m.: Nothing is scheduled. Time for their main meal.
- 3:00 p.m.: The second lamb is sacrificed, and the third hour of prayer begins.

If it took an hour to perform the sacrifices, followed by an hour of prayer, then they would have two free hours. One at 11:00 a.m. and one at 2:00 p.m. before tying up lambs at noon and 3:00 p.m. Both these eating windows fit nicely into the 17–7 intermittent fasting eating pattern as modeled in Exodus 16:21.

The Romance of Redemption

"Now Boaz said to her at mealtime, 'Come here, and eat of the bread, and dip your piece of bread in the vinegar.' So she sat beside the reapers, and he passed parched [grain] to her; and she ate and was satisfied, and kept some back. And when she rose up to glean, Boaz commanded his young men, saying, 'Let her glean even among the sheaves, and do not reproach her. Also let [grain] from the bundles fall purposely for her; leave [it] that she may glean, and do not rebuke her.' So she gleaned in the field until evening, and beat out what she had gleaned, and it was about an ephah of barley" (Ruth 2:14–17 NKJV).

The story of Ruth and Boaz paints a picture of a romantic story of redemption. Naomi was driven from her land representing Israel; Ruth was a non-Jew who was accepted into the family representing the church, and Boaz is the redeemer representing Christ Jesus (DeHaan 1970). While we are just going to look at a small portion of this story, I encourage everyone to read the entire book of Ruth in light of this picture. It's incredible.

But this area of scripture also gives us another glimpse of the time-restricted eating patterns found elsewhere in scripture. The wording here is very specific. We see that Boaz and Ruth are not just chatting it up snacking on some food, like budding relationships often do; rather, they were eating at "mealtime." A very specific time of day for the main meal to begin. They continued to eat until they were satisfied, and Ruth kept back some leftovers to take home to her mother-in-law, Naomi. Earlier in the story, we read that Boaz was well aware of what Ruth had done for her mother-in-law, when she had brought her back to her land and taken care of her after the death of Ruth's husband, Naomi's son. In return for Ruth's faithfulness, Boaz told Ruth to stay close to his young women and glean only in his field. Furthermore, he commanded his young men to purposefully let grain fall from the bundles as she gleaned in the field until evening.

Verse 17 tells us that Ruth gleaned about an ephah of barley. An ephah is a bushel of grain, which is approximately 35 liters or 145 cups. This clearly demonstrates that Ruth and Boaz needed to finish their meal well before evening, or she wouldn't have had the time needed to gather 145 cups of grain (just take a minute to imagine gathering 145 cups of grain from a field!). They would need to have finished their meal early in the afternoon around 3:00 p.m. to have the time necessary to glean.

Again, this story does not *prove* that Boaz and Ruth were following some God ordained eating pattern. However, what it clearly shows is Boaz's daily mealtime fits perfectly into the eating pattern God commanded the children of Israel to use while they were wandering in the wilderness just two generations prior. No doubt, the eating patterns established in the wilderness had continued to be passed down from generation to generation as the normal and customary practices.

Thus far, our studies have been taken out of the Old Testament. Let's now turn our focus to the New Testament. Do we see similar examples of the Exodus 16:21 eating pattern demonstrated in the New Testament as well? We sure do! As we will see in these next two well-known stories, the eating patterns have remained, but the times of those patterns have changed ever so slightly.

In the New Testament, we find Israel's eating pattern being changed by pushing the evening meal back a few hours—same eating pattern, just shifted a bit. We see evidence in the New Testament that points to meals being completed at the end of the day, around 4:00 to 6:00 p.m., followed by fifteen to seventeen hours of fasting before the next meal, including the famous "Breakfast by the Sea," being eaten between 9:00 and 11:00 a.m. the following day.

Passover Meal—The Lord's Supper

> So the disciples did as Jesus had directed them; and they prepared the Passover. When evening had come, He sat down with the twelve. (Matt. 26:19–20 NKJV)

> So His disciples went out, and came into the city, and found it just as He had said to them; and they prepared the Passover. In the evening He came with the twelve. (Mark 14:16–17 NKJV)

> When the hour had come, He sat down, and the twelve apostles with Him. Then He said to them, "With [fervent] desire I have desired to eat this Passover with you before I suffer; for I say to you, I will no longer eat of it until it is fulfilled in the kingdom of God." (Luke 22:14–16 NKJV)

> And supper being ended, the devil having already put it into the heart of Judas Iscariot, Simon's [son,] to betray Him, Jesus, knowing that the Father had given all things into His hands, and that He had come from God and was going to God, rose from supper and laid aside His garments, took a towel and girded Himself." (John 13:2–4 NKJV)

All three Gospels tell the account of the Passover Meal in their own distinct ways. Matthew and Mark each commented that the meal was to take place in the evening. Luke pointed out that it was at a predetermined hour just like the predetermined mealtime in which we saw Boaz and Ruth eat. But when we look at John's Gospel, we see a lot of additional details.

John records that suppertime had finished, and it was time for Jesus to start teaching His disciples their final lessons. In chapter 13, we see Jesus washing the disciples' feet as a picture of the cleansing that He would do for all of us when He conquered the grave. He identifies His betrayer, gives them a new commandment, and predicts Peter's denial. In chapter 14, we read that Jesus spoke that He was the way, the truth, and the life, as well as revealing that He and the Father are one, teaching them to ask and receive, and letting them know that He and the Father will dwell in us to give us peace.

In chapter 15, Jesus instructs His disciples that He is the True Vine, that the world will hate anyone who follows Him, and tells them the Holy Spirit will come when He is gone. In chapter 16, He explains that He had spoken these things so they would not stumble knowing that their message would be rejected by many Jews, as well as the Jewish leadership. He informs them how the Holy Spirit will be at work in them, that their sorrow of losing Him will turn to joy, and they will be scattered. "But be of good cheer; I have overcome the world."

He did all this *after* supper, and He wasn't even close to being finished. He still had to pray. John 18:1 tells us that after He had spoken, He and His disciples went to the garden to pray. And pray He did.

"Then they came to a place which was named Gethsemane; and He said to His disciples, 'Sit here while I pray'" (Mark 14:32 NKJV).

He went and prayed by Himself while His disciples were instructed to wait—not just once, but on several occasions. Jesus spent a lot of time praying, so much so that He found his disciples had fallen asleep.

> Then they came to a place which was named Gethsemane; and He said to His disciples, "Sit here while I pray." And He took Peter, James, and John with Him, and He began to be troubled and deeply distressed. Then He said to them, "My soul is exceedingly sorrowful, [even] to death. Stay here and watch." He went a little farther, and fell on the ground, and prayed that if it were possible, the hour might pass from Him. And He said, "Abba, Father, all things *are* possible for You. Take this cup away from Me; nevertheless, not what I will, but what You *will*." Then He came and found them sleeping, and said to Peter, "Simon, are you sleeping? Could you not watch one hour? "Watch and pray, lest you enter into temptation. The spirit indeed *is* willing, but the flesh *is* weak." Again, He went away and prayed, and spoke the same words. And when He returned, He found them asleep again, for their eyes were heavy; and they did not know what to answer Him. Then

He came the third time and said to them, "Are you still sleeping and resting? It is enough! The hour has come; behold, the Son of Man is being betrayed into the hands of sinners" (Mark 14:32–41 NKJV).

How long did the prayer time last? The text identifies at least three hours. The above three hours of prayer were not the only prayers recorded. Chapter 17 of John's Gospel records another lengthy prayer. Did He pray that prayer three times as recorded by Mark? Who knows? The text doesn't tell us. If Mark's account is any indication of Jesus's prayer time, then His time spent in prayer was significant. And why wouldn't it be? He had a lot to talk to the Father about. Things were about to get real—big time!

In John 17:1–26, John records a very lengthy prayer where Jesus first prayed for Himself in verses 1–5; He then prayed for His disciples in verses 6–19; and finished by praying for you and me in verses 20–26. I would encourage you to read John 17:1–26 in its entirety. The way Jesus taught us to pray in chapter 6 of Matthew's Gospel is often referred to as the Lord's Prayer. I would suggest to you that the *actual* Lord's Prayer is found in John's Gospel. A truly, beautiful petition to the Father.

The Gospels of Matthew and Mark clearly state that the Passover meal was to take place in the evening. The point we should take from the recording of such lengthy prayer times after the Passover meal is that the meal did not last well into the night; it couldn't have. As was customary, it ended early in the evening (Josephus VI. 9.3.). According to the recorded events that took place after their meal, there simply was not enough time. Scripture records lengthy in-depth conversations and teachings that were sure to last a fair amount of time. After an extensive and treasured time of study and instruction directly from the mouth of God Himself, Jesus then went to the garden and prayed. And He continued to pray, right up until the hour He was betrayed.

Jesus Breaks His Fast by the Sea of Galilee

"But when the morning had now come, Jesus stood on the shore; yet the disciples did not know that it was Jesus. Then Jesus said to them, "Children, have you any food?"

They answered Him, "No." And He said to them, "Cast the net on the right side of the boat, and you will find [some.]" So they cast, and now they were not able to draw it in because of the multitude of fish. Therefore that disciple whom Jesus loved said to Peter, "It is the Lord!" Now when Simon Peter heard that it was the Lord, he put on [his] outer garment (for he had removed it), and plunged into the sea. But the other disciples came in the little boat (for they were not far from land, but about two hundred cubits), dragging the net with fish. Then, as soon as they had come to land, they saw a fire of coals there, and fish laid on it, and bread. Jesus said to them, "Bring some of the fish which you have just caught." Simon Peter went up and dragged the net to land, full of large fish, 153; and although there were so many, the net was not broken. Jesus said to them, "Come [and] eat breakfast." Yet none of the disciples dared ask Him, "Who are You?"—knowing that it was the Lord. (John 21:4–12 NKJV)

Let's look at these passages a little closer. When Jesus asked the disciples if they had any food, the disciples did not recognize Him. After following His instructions to "cast the net on the right side of the boat," John shouted to Peter, "It is the Lord!" Peter immediately put on his garment and "plunged" into the sea swimming toward Jesus. The other disciples rowed the boat to shore to share some fish with them. The following scenario reveals that this *breakfast,* as we have always been taught, was actually a *brunch* fitting perfectly into the intermittent fasting pattern with that one slight change: the time at which the eating window would begin.

- The disciples fished all night and were in the boat when morning came.
- 7:00 a.m.: Not being recognized by the disciples, the resurrected Lord Jesus instructed them to cast their nets on the other side of the boat. They did so and struggled for some time unable to get all the fish into the boat because the multitude was so great.

- 8:00 a.m.: John recognized Jesus, and Peter jumped off the boat and swam two hundred cubits to shore. A cubit is about 18 inches in length, so Peter would have had to swim one hundred yards. The length of an entire football field.
- 9:00 a.m.: The other disciples get out of the big boat, into the small boat, and rowed one hundred yards to shore while dragging the 153 fish.
- 10:00 a.m.: Jesus had the fire going and was cooking fish. Jesus told them to bring some of the fish they had caught. Peter dragged the 153 large fish to land. They proceeded to clean, gut, debone, and prepare enough fish for all the disciples to eat.
- 11:00 a.m.: Jesus said, "Come, aristao with me," which is to take the *principal meal* of the day, or *to dine* according to *Strong's Concordance*. The Greek word was used three times in the New Testament, twice in the current context and once when Jesus dined in the afternoon with a Pharisee found in Luke 11:37. The translators used the word *breakfast* likely because of the context. However, when we observe the events as they took place, eating at midmorning is the more probable scenario rather than early in the morning. My Bible labels this account as "Breakfast by the Sea." And I would agree that they broke their fast by the sea all right, just not necessarily in the early morning. A better heading might be "Brunch by the Sea." It is likely that those involved in this story finished their evening meals between three and six o'clock the previous evening since it was the custom of first century Jews to have eaten their evening meals at the same hour they had their Passover meal (Whiston 1737). With all that took place as recorded by John in his gospel account, Jesus and the disciples would have fasted for fifteen hours if they ate between 7:00 and 9:00 a.m., fasted for sixteen hours if the meal was between 8:00 a.m. and 10:00 a.m., or fasted seventeen hours if they ate between 9:00 a.m. and 11:00 a.m. Before their meal at the shore, they would have flipped their metabolic switch about the time they recognized Jesus, causing them to be in a ketogenic state for three to five hours. More about flipping the switch and the ketogenic state to come.

Further Evidence of Time-Restricted Eating Patterns

> When Joseph saw Benjamin with them, he said to the
> steward of his house, "Take [these] men to my home, and
> slaughter an animal and make ready; for [these] men will
> dine with me *at noon*." (Gen. 43:16 NKJV)

> Then they made the present ready for Joseph's coming
> *at noon*, for they heard that they would eat bread there."
> (Gen. 43:25 NKJV)

Here we see two examples in Genesis where they ate at noon or
shortly thereafter. In the book of Samuel, we find another example of
their skipping breakfast.

> So the cook took up the thigh with its upper part and set
> [it] before Saul. And [Samuel] said, "Here it is, what was
> kept back. *It* was set apart for you. Eat; for until this time
> it has been kept for you, since I said I invited the people."
> So Saul ate with Samuel that day. When they had come
> down from the high place into the city, *Samuel* spoke with
> Saul on the top of the house. They arose early; and it was
> about the dawning of the day that Samuel called to Saul
> on the top of the house, saying, "Get up, that I may send
> you on your way." And Saul arose, and both went outside,
> he and Samuel. (1 Sam. 9:24–26 NKJV)

Here we see Saul and Samuel eating "that day." We also see them
arising "early" in the morning, with no mention of an early morning meal.
There are many places in scripture where the details are not mentioned.
In this case, however, the author records that they ate in the day, leading
us to believe that he would have recorded a very similar fact if they would
have eaten in the morning.

An Unveiling

God has revealed to us in His Word that we do not need to be constantly filled with food from morning 'til noon 'til night to maintain optimal health. He did not reveal any of this type of eating pattern in the Bible: nowhere. *He created* us to function best when we refrain from eating for a period of fifteen to seventeen hours a day and condense our eating into a seven- to nine-hour eating window. You will not find mention of an early morning meal that is blessed by God anywhere in the Bible. We see a late morning fish fry with Jesus in the New Testament; we see several examples of meals between noon and three, and we see examples of early evening meals, but never do we see meals in the morning. The only exception is when it is followed by a curse as was the case in the Golden Calf incident of Exodus 32.

In short, if you stop eating after your last meal of the day, either the afternoon or evening meal, skip breakfast, and start eating fifteen to seventeen hours later; after a few days, you will find that your energy, alertness, and mood will increase considerably. You will be putting your body in a position to heal itself, just as God designed it to, but with the added benefits of gradual weight loss, improved metabolic health, and an increased immunity from sickness and disease, as well as enjoying a higher quality of life.

The examples above are just a brief study of biblical eating patterns; however, in each case we see how time-restricted eating patterns are consistent with scripture in both the Old and New Testaments. Nowhere did we discover biblical eating patterns that consisted of three square meals a day, nor did we discover anywhere that one must have a hearty, stick to your ribs type breakfast every morning, knowing that after all, "it is the most important meal of the day." The truth is it just isn't.

Don't Be Too Dogmatic About It

Adopting the intermittent fasting patterns that God revealed in the Bible is not a commandment, nor is it necessary for salvation. I would argue that it is a good choice but still a choice. We see such eating patterns demonstrated throughout scripture, and now we have modern science revealing the benefits of such patterns. We saw in scripture that the Children of Israel were instructed to eat in this intermittent fasting pattern over three thousand years ago, and to emphasize the point, God had His children eat in this pattern for nearly half a century. He commanded it to them and gave them no choice. On the other hand, He does not command it to us, but He gives us a choice.

God did not reveal time-restricted eating patterns in the Bible because He wanted to take the joy out of our morning breakfasts or because He wanted to deny us the pleasure of a late-night snack; He revealed these eating patterns because He knows us and knows what is best for us. We are fearfully and wonderfully made (Ps. 139:13–14). Because *He skillfully formed our inward parts*, He knows exactly how to instruct us on our eating patterns for us to maximize the benefits. We simply need to trust that the way He trained His people, Israel, applies to all people. He wants to restore us daily, just as He restores all His creation. All we need do is eat *properly*.

Chapter 2

Optimized Health

Mystery of the Means

> "Before I began the study of medicine, I had become aware
> that most persons attacked by acute disease recovered, no
> matter how [they were] treated or by whom. It was often
> within the range of my knowledge that poor families
> living at a distance from physicians treated their sick, and
> at times, their severely sick with only "home remedies,"
> and I wondered over the mystery of means, [rather than]
> the mystery of the cure. (Edward Hooker Dewey, *The True
> Science of Living*)

In 1902, Dr. Edward Hooker Dewey was one of the few people in the
medical establishment who questioned the medical practices of the time.
During his twenty-eight-year career in the medical field, he witnessed
countless patients, many of whom he documented in his book, who were
in fact healed not by the established medical practices of stuffing the body
with food, alcohol ingestions, or forced feedings but rather by changing
their eating patterns. He would have his clients simply abstain from eating
after their last meal of the day until lunch the following day. We see his
personal breakthrough in the following excerpt:

> In the course of my human events I arose one morning
> in an unusual exhaustion from digestive taxing of an

evening meal that was not needed, and seated myself at a breakfast-table where the supply was adequate for a noon-meal at a farmhouse. For once I was not hungry. Why should I have been? I had only had the exercise called out in dressing since I retired [went to bed] the night before; but it had been thirteen hours since I had eaten my last meal, and not to eat until the next mealtime would involve an additional fast of five and a half [hours], in all eighteen hours and a half. Should I take the chances of going without a breakfast and be likely to faint dead away while trying to count some irregular pulse? Preposterous! ... I took my chances on a breakfast of coffee only, and so far from fainting during my forenoon ways, I had a forenoon of such lofty mental cheer, such energy of soul and body, such a sense of physical ease as I had not known since a young man in my later teens!

In the course of a few weeks there was such a quickening of my life in every line, that friends began to notice it." (Dewey 1894, 147–150)

Not only did he experience a favorable impact on his own mental and physical state, but Dewey also witnessed improvements on the effects of aging. The following story tells how a seventy-three-year-old obese woman had strikingly positive results. She had a constant cough, increasing deafness, was unable to go up and down stairs because of shortness of breath, and was limited as to when and where she could go on walks. It was her routine to have a light midmorning breakfast, a more substantial lunch at midday, a light evening meal, and an apple before bedtime: four daily meals (Dewey 1894, 131).

The meals were cut down to coffee in the morning, lunch at the usual time, a light evening meal, and no apple at bedtime. The improvements were immediate. In a few weeks, the cough went away, the deafness improved, the heart gained strength, and she began to decline in weight (ibid.). The following year, she was able to walk about the city and even found that she could walk up to half a mile up a decided grade. She often said that with the exception of getting up in age, "She has never felt in a general way any better in all her life." And now at the age of seventy-eight, "Her mind is as clear as crystal; and she is an enthusiast over the means whereby her life was saved and enlarged to a serener and more comfortable age." Unknowingly, she adopted the intermittent fasting eating pattern, resulting in an enriched life.

The *mystery* that Dr. Dewey discovered was the following: by eating in a time-restricted eating pattern, you could optimize your health by simply changing the time of when you would eat. The empirical evidence that he himself experienced was substantial, observable, repeatable, and consistent. He began to advise patients suffering from overtaxed stomachs to abandon all food in the morning except for "that cup that cheers." This practice was considered recklessly dangerous and was contrary to the established medical practices of his day. Nonetheless, his advice was found to be "absolutely safe" (ibid., 150).

But *how* did it work? What was the means? He understood the who, what, when, and where. His *skipping breakfast* treatment clearly worked, but the question as to *why* it worked forever eluded him. Could scientific evidence ever exist that would be accepted by the established medical community? Was that type of proof even attainable? Clearly, Dr. Dewey's results were irrefutable, but evidence could not be proven in the laboratory. At least not yet.

Fast-forward 120 years, and we get to the research done by Dr. Mark Mattson. Dr. Mattson is currently the adjunct professor of Neuroscience at Johns Hopkins University and was previously chief of the Laboratory of Neurosciences at the National Institute on Aging. Mattson has pioneered research uncovering the way the brain responds to fasting and exercise. During his thirty-plus years of research, he discovered how intermittent fasting slows the effects of aging and reduces the risk of diseases—including obesity and Alzheimer's disease—while improving both brain and body performance (Mattson 2022). His research reveals that, in most cases, the body can recover if we would simply adopt the eating patterns as outlined in his book *The Intermittent Fasting Revolution*. The benefits of adopting such patterns will result in optimal mental health and enhanced physical performance, much like we saw with Dewey's research.

We are about to take up a comparison of the scientific evidence provided from Dr. Dewey's fieldwork in the nineteenth century with Dr. Mattson's laboratory research in the twenty-first century. We will contrast the research tools available to each doctor, and we will find that both men were onto something that *should have* or *could have* the power to change how we view medicine and time-restricted eating patterns.

Flipping the Switch

I was recently speaking with a good friend of mine about my excitement over discovering Mattson's new book on intermittent fasting. The concepts and conclusions were spelled out so clearly and concisely that, much to my surprise, I was able to explain the benefits of the eating pattern as laid out in the book having only gotten through the introduction. The introduction alone was so "to the point" that I was able to understand how the body was able to produce and burn ketones from fat cells.

As Mattson explains, the process of ketone production begins twelve hours after your last meal (or energy intake), defining energy intake as ingesting anything containing calories. Mattson outlines this amazingly simple concept, which transitions into an equally amazing complex metabolic process. This essential fat-burning process occurs when your body undergoes what he has labeled as "flipping the metabolic switch." That's it. It's that simple. Just get in the habit of flipping your metabolic switch on a regular basis. Once you have abstained from caloric intake for twelve hours, enabling your body to flip its metabolic switch, you should stay in that condition for as long as you would like in order to maximize the overall health benefits.

Dewey also observed that there is a time when your body creates what he called "rich blood" after a time of fasting (Dewey 1894, 176, 180). When one abstains from eating after the evening meal until lunch the following day, the body will in effect flip the metabolic switch and create such rich blood. We would later discover this to be a phenomenon synonymous with ketone production. A ketone is an organic molecule that enters the bloodstream immediately after it is created and has the same energy found in glucose. The benefit is that it has far fewer free radicals, which has the effect of removing damaged molecules from your body (Mattson 2022, 102).

Ketogenic State

Mattson discovered that your liver stores 400 to 500 calories of glucose (energy) after eating. When the glucose is depleted in a fasted state, your fat cells convert to ketones, which your body uses as fuel rather than the glucose that *was* stored in your liver. As previously discussed, this process takes place approximately twelve hours after your last meal (energy intake). Your body then undergoes the *metabolic switch* whereby it creates ketones, produced from fat, which are immediately transmitted into the bloodstream (Mattson 2022). Not only is your body burning excess fat as fuel, but it is also using the ketones to produce many additional mental and physiological benefits. (If you're interested in more of the science surrounding intermittent fasting, I would suggest picking up Mattson's book.)

Both Mattson and Dewey discovered the benefits of adopting time-restricted eating patterns during their respective research. Mattson, through scientific laboratory studies at Johns Hopkins University, proved that after twelve hours of fasting the body would create the molecules necessary to get into what he refers to as a ketogenic state. Dewey, from personal experience and through his fieldwork and empirical evidence witnessed from his patients during the late 1800s, theorized that by not eating for thirteen to eighteen hours, your body would create that self-healing rich blood. While their language and means may have differed, both men were correct. Dewey's findings in the nineteenth century have been validated by Dr. Mattson's work in the twenty-first century. As a result of these two pioneers researching the topic for more than sixty years (combined), within two different millennia, the God-given mystery of good health has been solved.

The Benefits of Intermittent Fasting

One of the conclusions resulting from both Dewey's and Mattson's research was that adopting an intermittent fasting eating pattern slows the effects of aging. The question then becomes, "Does slowing the effects of aging mean that we will *live* longer?" The answer is, "Well ... sort of."

When you consider the fact that we are less likely to die from age-related ailments such as stroke, type 2 diabetes, Alzheimer's disease, etc., then the answer to the question is an emphatic Yes! We will absolutely live longer but not because the length of our average life expectancies are expected to increase. Rather we will live longer because we will have reduced our risk of contracting debilitating and deadly diseases. According to both Dewey and Mattson, adopting an intermittent fasting time-restricted eating pattern will most certainly result in an increased quality of life, both for us *and* for those around us.

Many of us suffer from excessive abdominal fat, which puts us at-risk for additional health concerns. A leading cause for this excessive fat arises from an overindulgent, sedentary lifestyle resulting in caloric intake in excess of caloric expenditures. Granted, sometimes it is merely genetics or other factors, and many of us spend years trying to "crack the weight loss code," if you will. But Mattson's extensive research and study on the topic demonstrates that excessive belly fat can be reduced simply by putting our bodies into a ketogenic state on a regular basis. Additionally, the benefits are not limited to weight loss. In fact, his research revealed that many neurological, as well as physiological, benefits result as well. The list includes but is not limited to the following benefits:

- reducing the risk of the onset of Alzheimer's disease;
- reducing the risk of the onset of Parkinson's disease;
- improving metabolism by means of a metabolic switch where your body produces ketones from fat;
- reducing obesity and type II diabetes;
- cardiovascular improvements, which reduce the chances of stroke;
- reduction of infectious diseases;
- reduction in some forms of cancer;
- Increased mental acuity;
- reducing the disease related effects of aging;
- reduction of inflammation;
- and if that's not enough for you men, you will experience an increase in cyclic GMP, which results in an increase in sildenafil (more commonly known as Viagra) (Mattson 2022, 123).

It may seem too good to be true, but that is precisely what the science proves despite most physicians' propensity to medicate for nearly every diagnosis. If one adopts time-restricted eating patterns (intermittent fasting), over time they will find that their need for prescription drugs is reduced drastically. Additionally, their mental acuity and weight stabilization are sure to improve. All these findings are in chapters 2 and 3 of Mattson's book as well as throughout part II of Dewey's.

Slowing the Effects of Aging—Forty-Four Is the New Thirty-Three

Many of us have heard the phrase that forty is the new thirty, meaning people in their forties feel as physically fit and active as they did in their thirties. That certainly holds true when considering the effects of two great NFL quarterbacks as well. As of the writing of this book, it was the year 2022, and Tom Brady just re-signed with the Tampa Bay Buccaneers. He was selected to the Pro-Bowl at age forty-four and won the Superbowl at age forty-three. Also in the year 2022, the Denver Broncos traded for Pro-Bowl quarterback Russel Wilson and signed him to a seven-year deal worth $296 million! He was thirty-three years old at the time and said he wanted to play ten to thirteen more years in Denver. It is incredible how these professional athletes have been able to defy the aging process. One of them already has, and another expects to lengthen his football career. Both Brady and Wilson are world-class athletes operating at the top of their games. They have been gifted with God-given natural talents and good mental and physical health.

Are *we*, like these professional athletes, able to limit the effects of aging? If we have the understanding and awareness to eat in Intermittent fasting patterns, the answer is yes. God created humankind perfectly to be able to live in harmony within his or her surroundings forever, but because we are not perfect, we find ourselves living in a world that has been corrupted by sin. Most of us are familiar with the story of Adam and Eve eating what was at that time forbidden fruit. When Adam and Eve took a bite out of the apple, sin forever entered God's perfect creation, which is to say that we are now unable to fully enjoy our bodies in the way God created them to function. As a matter of fact, when sin entered our world, creation suffered the effects. Weeds, thorns, thistles, earthquakes, storms, and the like are now part of our world. Not only was paradise lost, but our ability to live in perfectly created bodies was lost as well.

Nevertheless, God, in His foreknowledge and love for us, already established a work-around. He knew we would sin, or miss the mark, so He sent His Son as a substitutionary atonement to take care of that sin once and for all. In His foreknowledge He knows the many mistakes we are going to make along the way in our walk with Him. That's why He had the solution to all life's problems written in advance in the Bible. If we live our lives on that foundation, nothing can bring us down—at least not permanently. The same holds true with our health. The key to good health can be attained simply by modifying our eating patterns to align with the eating patterns as demonstrated in the Bible. By doing so, we can slow the harmful effects of aging. We may not have multiple Superbowl rings or be able to zip a forty-yard pass over the middle, but we are going to feel great and be able to fulfill all the things that God created us to do, *for Him.*

Chapter 3

Finely Sculpted of Divinely Tuned?

As I mentioned earlier in the book, Mattson and Dewey discovered the same phenomenon yet attributed their astounding findings to two very different sources—polar opposites, you might say. According to Mattson, our ability to fight disease and recover from illness is a result of our finely "sculpted" bodies but not sculpted by who you might think. Rather, he states, "As you will discover in this book, evolution has "sculpted" our cells and organ systems such that they respond to intermittent fasting in ways that enable them to function optimally" (Mattson 2022). Sculpting connotes a sculptor much like design speaks of a designer. There's an act of cause and effect in play here. We are living proof of the effect, and Matson's and Dewey's research prove what amazing bodies we have. But who or what made it all come to pass (pardon the pun)? Clearly there was a force at work in the creation of our miraculous bodies. But what was it? What was the cause?

Many believe, as does Mattson, that evolution "sculpted" our bodies to the refined level of sophistication that we enjoy today. Darwinian evolutionists believe our existence is the result of random chance, and it is only *because of this lucky break* that life on earth exists at all. They believe matter is the only thing that has or will ever exist, and therefore, there is no reason for a greater purpose or for the very existence of human life. It just is. Thankfully, just as Dewey recognized, we too are learning this position is far from the truth and completely off target with reality. As we shall discover as did Pink Floyd in the seventies, "Wrong! Do it again! If you don't eat your meat, you can't have any pudding. How can you have any pudding if you don't eat your meat?" (Waters 1979). As we will see, the proof is in the pudding, not the primordial soup.

So You're Telling Me there's a Chance.

The growing scientific enigma is that just as the odds of Lloyd scoring a date with Mary in the movie *Dumb and Dumber was exceedingly small,* science has now revealed that the odds of our existence on this planet, at this time, in this universe, under these perfect conditions, are *infinitesimally small* (Metaxas 2021). Given random chance and luck over billions of years, we should not be here; but we are. Not only do we exist, but we exist in a finely tuned and masterfully created universe as well as in finely tuned and masterfully created bodies.

Accepting the notion that we came from a cosmic accident that fell into place by chance resulting in billions of years of evolution, despite that all observable geological evidence and natural laws of science say otherwise. And accepting a theory, taught as fact, that we progressed by natural selection using a life-killing process called survival of the fittest. All the while, asserting that matter evolved so precisely over those billions of years by learning to identify and separate good cells from bad ones by means of the garbage disposal process known as autophagy. And this resulting in nonlife springing into life in our human cells and evolving to the meticulous level in which we now find ourselves seems a bit of a stretch, to say the least. Boy are we lucky—luckier than Lloyd.

Through this process of autophagy (self-eating), our sculpted bodies can identify bad cells, which are promptly killed off by good cells. According to Professor Mattson, this process can be aided by the time-restricted eating patterns that we were forced to use ages ago when we—Neanderthals— would hunt and gather food.

Many Christians would agree with the theory of evolution, but they would qualify their belief by asserting that God had His hand in the process by putting all matter, then life, into existence; He then *tipped the domino* by which our bodies evolved into the finely tuned state of existence that we enjoy today. Theistic evolutionists would say that our body's ability to self-regulate is a God-given quality and that God created us using the process of evolution.

I Know It's Not Very Woke, but Can We Simply Agree to Disagree?

As a Creationist, my position asserts that our finely tuned bodies have existed from the moment at which God spoke Adam into being. We Creationists believe that we were made perfectly in every way, just like the rest of God's handiwork including plant life, animal life, and human life. This was the age that biblical scholars refer to as the *Age of Innocence*. That is, sin had yet to enter God's creation. Everything that God had shaped on earth existed in a perfect state in perfect harmony where all life was thriving. The metabolic health of His creation was working as planned, and humankind was free to eat whatever plant life pleased them save the one forbidden fruit.

So while it may not be very "woke," I simply can't agree that our bodies miraculously evolved into the incredible and finely tuned forms we have today. You will see for yourself how "chance" did not get us to where we are today but instead that we are the intentional act of an all-knowing and all-loving God.

A Defensive Genius

We've all heard the phrases "defense wins championships," or, in the worst-case scenario, "you'd better have a plan B." Well, as it turns out, God already knew Adam and Eve were going to eat the fruit of the forbidden tree. They were permitted to eat anything they pleased except that infamous fruit. It was hanging from the tree of the knowledge of good and evil, and the serpent had convinced them that if they ate from it, they would not surely die. The opposite would be true. Being deceived, Eve saw that the tree was good for food, was pleasant to the eyes, and was desirable to make one wise, so, what the heck? Bon appétit! Dig in! Both Adam and Eve disobeyed God.

Not to worry though, God had already put a perfect solution in place. As we saw earlier, God in His foreknowledge knew Adam and Eve would sin, but what we didn't know was that He had already created the solution. He was going to send His Son, the second person of the trinity, and the same person who was with God before the foundation of the world (John 17:5). In addition, because of humankind's propensity to miss the mark, He subsequently put Cherubim (guardian angels) in place to guard the tree of life. If they ate from the tree of life, they would live forever in a fallen state (Gen. 3:22–24). Adam's and Eve's deaths were an act of mercy. To live forever in a fallen state would have resulted in eternal separation between God and His creation. That's not gonna happen; God would have none of it! Instead, He would send His Son to enable a perfect God to dwell with an imperfect humankind forever. Adam and Eve would be saved by the Messiah to come, just as we are saved by the Messiah who conquered death. If that's a plan B, I'll take it!

God, in His infinite wisdom, planned to send His son to take care of our sin problem and to save our souls. But He also created a food source by which He built a natural defense mechanism to enable our physical bodies to optimize our health in this fallen state. His defensive game-plan included many things. One of which came in the form of a highly concentrated noxious phytochemical that would be lethal to all animal life should they eat it. According to Mattson, "phytochemicals functioned as 'antifeedants' deterring insects, herbivores, and omnivores from eating them," which would give humans the ability to consume such plants

(Mattson 2022, 48, 155–59). How awesome is that? Our Creator knew we would end up in a fallen state, so before He even created us, He put into place an ecosystem able to sustain us in that state.

Mattson's research identified four major defense mechanisms. They can be found in both our bodies and in plant life. God created what is known today as phytochemicals, as mentioned in the previous paragraph. These chemicals enable both animal life and human life to have an ample supply of nutrient rich foods. The first defense mechanism is the fact that concentrated levels of phytochemicals have a very bitter taste. This taste is found in the buds, the skin, the seeds, and roots of certain foods. Take fruit for example. "As fruit ripens, the concentration of phytochemicals in the skin and seeds dissipate over time making them palatable" (ibid.). As an example, just think of unripe peaches or plums. The bitterness deterring you from eating an unripe fruit is all due to phytochemicals!

The second defense mechanism against overconsumption is simply to vomit, which is self-explanatory given that your body will not retain things not intended to be consumed. The third mechanism involves *enzymes* in our livers that degrade or modify the phytochemicals. This chemical degradation occurs within ten minutes to an hour with the benefit of eliminating the accumulation and concentration of the noxious chemicals. Because plants, animals, and humans were created to coexist, God created animals without the liver enzymes needed to perform the function that human bodies perform; thus, deterring them from overindulging on man's food source.

The fourth defense mechanism is a result of our bodies having been created with a natural stress response system known as hormesis. Hormesis is a dose-response phenomenon where our bodies can adapt to *some* toxic chemicals. While at high doses they produce harmful biological effects, at low doses the exact same thing will produce beneficial effects (Mattson 2022, 106, 158, 160). I liken hormesis to the first bite of a funnel cake; the initial bite tastes oh-so good—boost of energy and a little serotonin—but as the dose increases, watch out, the effects become very detrimental often times resulting in a sick stomach.

> And as for you, be fruitful and multiply; Bring forth abundantly in the earth and multiply in it. (Gen. 9:7 NKJV)

Whether it be by theistic evolution, or by the miracle of God's finely tuned creation, humans and animals have coexisted from earth's beginning. Adam and Eve were created by God and were free to enjoy all of God's creation. This act of creation is evidence of God's perfect love for us. We find noxious phytochemicals in nutrient rich plants, fruits, and vegetables to protect those plants (Mattson 2022, 156–57) so that humankind could freely enjoy the richness of His creation.

Just imagine it. God created the biggest, most wonderful all-you-can-eat salad bar—the lettuce would never wilt, nor would it run out of your favorite ingredients. Everything about it was perfect. He also created humankind with free will and it is *because* of this free will that we can express our genuine love for Him. If He *did not* give us this freedom and merely created us as some sort of human robots programmed to love Him no matter the circumstance, there would be no evidence of this love. How could we know that our love was genuine if we had no say in the matter? Therefore, God gave us the choice of obeying Him or not, so we could experience the richness of His love.

In His perfect wisdom, God knew the enemy would work tirelessly to corrupt His creation. He allowed sin to slither into the world when He gave Adam and Eve the freedom of choosing whether or not to eat of the forbidden fruit. Before the fall of humankind had even happened, God put in place natural defense mechanisms, some of which were mentioned previously, throughout His earth, so His creation could thrive. His plan all along was for the *entire* world to be saved. Not just the Jews, but everyone! Genius!

Life from Nonlife … *Really*?

The debate between evolutionism and creationism has raged on for ages and will, no doubt, continue to do so until the Lord returns. However, both evolutionist and creationist are faced with the same dilemma of when life began. Both camps must define the very first source of life if they are going to have a strong position. *What* was the origin? *When* did it begin? *Who or what* was the trigger? *How* did inorganic matter become a living organism? *How* did that first cell learn to split itself in two and evolve into a fish, grow legs, walk, and fly while enduring the survival of the fittest test required of the evolutionary process? That's a pretty big question to merely take at face value, thus it deserves to be questioned.

So the question becomes, were we *created beings*, or did we emerge from some prebiotic primordial soup where nonlife suddenly sprang into life by means of a cosmic lightning strike as science alleges? Science just doesn't know. Many claim they know, but they have not been intellectually honest enough to admit that their accepted belief in materialistic evolution fails to hold up to the scientific evidence and the scientific method. They have accepted the theory of evolution as fact since it was accepted as fact by their contemporaries years before. This is the same type of practice the Pharisees were using when Jesus called them hypocrites a couple thousand years ago. They honored Jesus with their lips, but their hearts were far from them (Mark 7:5–7). Science claims nonlife became life absent a creator, but their hearts are not in it. They just can't admit it.

As time goes by and new science is revealed, we see the science is slowly concluding that the many things spoken of as fact in the Bible are proving to be true scientifically as well. The more discoveries that are made, the more artifacts unearthed, the more clinical research that is conducted, all point in the direction of science confirming what the Bible has claimed all along: the truth.

A modern example of science catching up with biblical claims is evidenced by the invention of the Hubble telescope. Since its advancement in the 1940s, the vast majority of scientists now agree that the universe is expanding. If it is expanding, then it had to have a starting point. No longer do scientists believe the, once accepted as fact, conclusion that matter in the universe is, and always will be, a constant. This concept had been shattered. The Hubble telescope and others like it prove that the universe is expanding. In fact, Dr. Collins, a physician-geneticist, says the universe is flying apart.

"If everything in the universe is flying apart, reversing the arrow of time would predict that at some point these galaxies were together in one incredibly massive entity. Hubble's observations started a deluge of experimental measurements that over the last seventy years have led to the conclusion by the vast majority of physicists and cosmologists that the universe began at a single moment; *now* commonly referred to as the Big Bang" (Collins 2006, 64).

Many believe the universe is billions of years old containing a "young earth." Others believe the Earth is just over six thousand years old. This mystery is something that cannot be proven definitively in scripture. Dr. Arnold Fruchtenbaum in his commentary on Genesis explores three common theories of creation. The initial chaotic theory, pre-creation chaos theory, and the gap or restoration theory (Fruchtenbaum 23–26). All three are interesting, and I'd encourage that you read Fruchtenbaum's work if you want more information, but we must keep in mind these are just theories. In this book, we will stick to interpretations known as fact found in scripture.

Evolutionism and creationism have been at odds with each other for years. I would submit, as did Dr. Dewey with the medical practices of his time, that science is still in the process of uncovering the mysteries of the universe.

In the early 1900s, German meteorologist Alfred Wegener proposed a theory of continental drift for a supercontinent he called Pangea. Discovering Pangea birthed the idea that the original earth was once a single massive continent that drifted apart (look at any world map, and you will see how the puzzle fits). His ideas were too radical at the time and largely rejected until the evidence of continental drift was accumulated in the 1960s (Clarey 2020, 117, 120). Then God said, "Let the waters under the heavens be gathered together into one place, and let the dry land appear; and it was so (Gen. 1:9).

The reality is that the accepted *scientific facts* of one hundred years ago would seem primitive by today's standards. Likewise, it is reasonable to expect that the accepted *scientific facts* of today will seem primitive one hundred years from now. Since the scientific community has been less than honest with the origin of life by slipping evolution into the prelife conversation, who's to say they have not used this sort of sleight of hand in determining the age of our universe? We just don't know.

Physics relies on what is known as the cosmological principle to determine the age of the universe. This principle stands on the idea that the universe is both "homogenous" and "isotropic"—that is, all forces are expected to act uniformly throughout the entire universe in all directions.

Is this principle an absolute? It is if you want to date the age of the universe at its current rate of expansion. But if this principle is not absolute, all bets are off. Could it be that at the time of creation the universe was expanding at a much more rapid pace, and has since slowed significantly? If other scientific assumptions have been proven false, there seems to be reason for questioning the validity of the cosmological principle. There is only one source that offers up a solution that has not and never will change. It is the only source that has and will remain constant forever—God's Word. The Bible has proven repeatedly that it is the infallible, inerrant Word of God, and the more we learn, the more we study, and the more we seek to understand, the more we see clearly.

May I Interest Anyone in a Game of Horseshoes?

Growing up, I often played horseshoes in the backyard with my friends. Those of you familiar with the game know that when you get a ringer—that is, when both ends of the shoe are past the post, you score three points. If you get a horseshoe within one horseshoe's length of the post, you get two points. If you get a leaner—the shoe is leaning against the post—you score one point. If you have neither, but you stayed within the foul lines and had a horseshoe closer than your competitor, you get one point. There are many ways to score in this game. One of which is to simply get closer to the target than your opponent. You've probably heard the saying *"getting close* only counts in horseshoes and hand grenades." When measured with the scientific method, just getting close doesn't cut the mustard, or at least it shouldn't.

The more we learn, the more we discover, the more science advances, one thing is becoming increasingly clear. The scientific evidence necessary to support abiogenesis (the leap from nonlife to life) is proving to be a mathematical impossibility. According to one of the world's most renowned nanoscientists, James Tour, when questioned on whether life could have emerged randomly from nonlife some four billion years ago, says emphatically, "based on what we now know, the idea is undeniably preposterous." He goes on to say, "The real problem is that scientists are mostly too stubborn to admit this, and what they are purporting to show (nonlife springing to life) can never actually be shown." We now know, having tried and failed and tried and failed over and over for the past seventy years, is how truly ignorant we are on the subject. "It cannot ever happen," he says (Metaxas 2021, 100). Never means never. They may have gotten close, but they are fudging it. Horseshoes anyone?

The scientific method requires all theories to be peer reviewed, be proven, and be repeatable, preferably many times by many scientists. In 1952, two University of Chicago scientists conducted a study known as the Miller-Urey experiment. In this so-called experiment, they claimed to have created what they theorized was a pool of water filled with a cocktail of four simple chemicals with the goal of approximating some prebiotic soup that they theorized existed before life existed. Their conclusion was that life came into existence from nonlife when a cosmic lightning strike hit the soup. Now the only thing left for science to do was to repeat the experiment. Because that's what science does, right? At least that is what the scientific method requires for an experiment to be known as "scientific."

Recall when nanoscientist James Tour said "it could not ever happen"? Despite their most heroic efforts for more than seventy years, the scientific community has tried and failed, tried and failed over and over again to substantiate these claims. These failures have proven consistent over time despite their having every motivation to succeed. Dr. Francis Collins, in his book *The Language of God,* asks the question, "How did self-replicating organisms arise in the first place? It is fair to say that at this present time, we simply do not know." Collins continues, "Despite substantial effort by multiple investigators, however, the basic building blocks of RNA, has not been achievable in a Miller-Urey type of experiment, nor has a fully self-replicating RNA been possible to design" (Collins 2006, 90, 91). The scientific community claims there is evidence of life emerging from nonlife; however, it has never been proven, much less repeated. As Eric Metaxas would say, in his famously articulate Ivy League style, "How embarrassing."

Now we see clearly that abiogenesis is *not* scientific. The scientific method requires an experiment to be observable and repeatable. In the case of Stanley Miller and Harold Urey, they were the only two scientists to make such a claim, and it remains an impossible experiment to perform, much less repeat. So that leads to a very valid question. Why has the scientific community accepted as scientific fact the claim that life sprang from nonlife by random chance? I'll leave that answer up to Mr. Eric Metaxas. "Can it be that everyone has been trained to nod in agreement at the concept of evolution, so that if we sneak it into this conversation of abiogenesis *(nonlife becoming life)* we can pretend that evolution extends everywhere, including into the world before life ... Why would anyone use the term 'evolution' in a definition of abiogenesis, except because their materialist ideology is more important than truth and clarity?" (Metaxas 2021, 115).

You Can't *Handle* the Truth!

Remember in the 1993 movie *A Few Good Men* when the young Lieutenant Kaffee interrogated the more seasoned Colonel Nathan Jessup imploring him to tell the truth? The colonel emphatically responded, "You can't *handle* the truth!" We see something very similar in this instance. Just as the colonel believed the lieutenant was unable to accept or handle the reality of what he was about to reveal, as science progresses, it is becoming more and more clear that the Darwinian evolutionism camp is either unwilling or unable to accept the truth. The truth is that nonlife evolving into life is a fabricated myth. As James Tour said, "They are fudging it."

The materialistic Darwinian view of evolution stands in stark opposition to the universally accepted scientific laws of thermodynamics. The first law of thermodynamics deduces that energy can neither be created nor destroyed. That begs the question: Where did it come from in the first place? What exploded? The second law of thermodynamics is where we find the concept known as entropy.

Entropy is the scientific fact that, over time, everything tends toward randomness and disorder. Things become disarrayed over time, not assembled as some would like to assert. Over time things become more and more disorderly, not more and more orderly. Every scientist on the planet would agree, and yet they deftly assert something quite the opposite when they sneak evolution into the prelife argument. They have been doing so for years.

The evidence seems to be pointing us in the direction that we are human beings with finely-tuned bodies created by God in His own image. The idea that nonlife sprung into life absent a Creator is simply not possible. We have been created *with*, and *for*, a purpose: *His* purpose. We are *not* the result of randomly connected matter that came to life when some primordial, prebiotic soup was struck by lightning 3.8 billion years ago, predated by a big bang that happened by accident ten billion years earlier. Where's the hope in that? *Exactly*, there *is* no hope. It appears science has been so influenced by the cultural narrative of the day stating that science and faith cannot coexist. Well, they can, and they do. In fact, the more we know, the more it's proven true. No longer should we accept the narrative that we are a product of Darwinian evolution and that we exist for no reason at all. No longer should we just believe what atheists and materialists tell us to believe.

The truth is that we have been fearfully and wonderfully made by God in His own image. This fact was evidenced in part by Dr. Dewey's empirical evidence conducted over 120 years ago and is supported by Dr. Mattson's extensive scientific research conducted in the here and now of the twenty-first century. The scientific community has been unable to reproduce their beloved Miller/Urey experiment despite billions of dollars spent trying to do so. Materialists, and for that matter, much of the scientific community, are not prepared for the consequences of allowing such views to take hold. To do so would be an admission, in part, that there is a Creator-God. Things are beginning to become much clearer.

Just as the seasoned Colonel Jessup retorted to young Lieutenant Kaffee, "You can't handle the truth!" Well, neither can they, or so it seems.

The Mystery of the Cure
Eating Pattern

I am reminded of another 1990s movie. This one being the 1993 hit *Kindergarten Cop*. In one scene, Arnold Schwarzenegger answers a question from a student when the student asks, "What's the matter?"

Schwarzenegger replies, "I have a headache."

"It might be a tumor," the student responds.

To which Schwarzenegger unequivocally says, *"It's not a tuma! ...* It's not a tuma at all."

In the movie, Schwarzenegger was playing the role of a police officer (cop) who was posing as a kindergarten teacher to apprehend a criminal. As evidenced by this and other scenes, he was not a very good teacher. Not a good teacher *at all*.

When I was considering a name for my newly discovered time-restricted eating pattern, I was tempted to call it, "The Daily Cure Diet." After all, by following this pattern *daily* our bodies will frequently get into a ketogenic state, optimize overall health with the added benefit of burning fat resulting in weight loss. All we *need* to do is follow the intermittent fasting patterns God demonstrates in the Bible that just so happen to be identical to intermittent fasting patterns that are so popular today and that are proven by science to be effective.

But then, just as Schwarzenegger was frustrated with the timing of the student's question, I was frustrated with the direction I was going with the benefits that result from adopting these eating patterns. I, too, was way off the mark. Mattson and Dewey clearly did not see daily fasting as a diet; and they too could state unequivocally, "It's not a diet! It's not a diet *at all*." Instead, it's an eating pattern designed to optimize overall health and slow the effects of aging. And what the heck, you might even lose a couple a pounds!

Skeptics might argue, "Wait a minute, the dictionary defines the word diet as a "regimen of eating to reduce one's weight," so it actually *is* a diet for weight loss." To which I would respond, I agree, in part. The common vernacular of the day uses the word *diet* as the type of regimen to reduce one's weight. But it is also defined as "food and drink regularly consumed" and "habitual nourishment" (*Webster's Dictionary*).

It's not a strict regimen of eating (or dieting as we commonly refer) to reduce one's weight. More accurately, it is a form of *habitual nourishment* with an emphasis on the time frame when nourishment is to be consumed. Instead of continuing our common eating pattern of breakfast, snack, lunch, dinner, followed by dessert, we need to adopt a time-restricted eating pattern to enable our bodies to optimize our overall health and performance the way God intended.

After searching scripture, I am convinced now more than ever that this method of eating should be modeled after the time-restricted eating patterns we find in the Bible. An example of a 16/8 eating pattern would look something like the following:

- 7:00 p.m.—Finish your last meal of the day.
- 7:00 a.m.—Your body undergoes a metabolic switch whereby it starts burning fat to create ketones.
- 11:00 a.m.—Your body has been in a ketogenic state for four hours: time for lunch—a moderate lunch. Remember, because you are inside your eating window, snacks are permissible. Preferably you chose healthy snacks such as nuts, fruit, yogurt, eggs. Sugars

and processed foods should be consumed in moderation and definitely nothing deep-fried.

- 7:00 p.m.—You've completed your evening meal. It's time to start fasting to get into that ketogenic state tomorrow morning.

Three of the time-restricted eating patterns Dr. Mattson puts forth in his book are 15/9, 16/8, or 17/7 fasts. These patterns include a lengthy fast, followed by a shorter eating window. A 16/8 intermittent fasting pattern was shown above (see the last few pages of this book for a simple outline of a daily eating pattern that can be used as a reference). By using the above model, you are flipping your metabolic switch at 7:00 a.m., which means your body will have been in a ketogenic state for a full four hours, reaping *all* the benefits that come with it.

You may choose any pattern that fits your lifestyle. If you work evenings, you may consider adjusting the pattern by several hours. The key is to deplete the glucose stored in your liver over a twelve-hour period by not taking in any energy (calories), which will enable your body to flip the metabolic switch to create ketones. You may want to start more slowly by using the 15/9 pattern and work your way up to a 16/8 or even a 17/7. All the patterns will get you into the much-desired and beneficial ketogenic state. The longer you remain in that state, the better the outcome and greater the benefits (Mattson 2022).

If you find that a seventeen-hour fast is too much for you, as I mentioned, start with only fifteen or sixteen hours. You will still have the benefit of being in a full ketogenic state for three to four hours each day. This is still an extremely good place to be. After your last meal, stick with sugar-free liquids such as water, sugar-free soft drinks, and the like. The following morning you *will* want to start your day with water, black coffee, or tea with no cream or sugar. The key is no energy intake (anything containing calories) until you are ready to break your fast. Juices are really great in the morning, I know. But the ketone energy rush you will get to experience by skipping the juice and enabling those ketones to rush through your bloodstream is well worth the sacrifice.

Breakfast: "*That Vulgar Habit*"

In the introduction of Dewey's book, Reverend George Pentecost's son, who was a great devotee of his breakfast, adopted what he saw as a new, most sensible theory of living and gave up his most beloved breakfast. (The introduction is so telling that I included a complete copy, which can be found in Appendix 2.) Because of the positive results he experienced, "He now playfully speaks of breakfast to his friends as, that vulgar habit." After finishing your last meal of the day, you would do well to *avoid eating anything* until lunch, including that vulgar habit.

If you believe, like many, that you will lack the protein and energy necessary to sustain yourself throughout the morning, you are mistaken. On the contrary, with a little discipline and self-awareness, you will be able to rid yourself of the routine of breaking your fast first thing in the morning, and you will begin embracing this new routine. Having your first meal around midday will become the norm, and you will come to love it! Your energy levels, as well as your stamina, are sure to rise (Dewey 1894).

Surprised by Joy

No, I'm not going to give you an excerpt from C. S. Lewis's scholarly autobiography *Surprised by Joy* (you should be so lucky); rather, I am going to explain the feeling that will come upon you, most unexpectedly, when you adopt an intermittent eating pattern lifestyle. As you approach the time to break your fast—much to your surprise—you are going to find that you have more mental acuity, as well as more energy, than you would have had if there had been a meal churning in your stomach. You will find your metabolic heart rate has kicked into high gear, and you are going to be thinking with increased clarity. As an unanticipated benefit, you are going to experience gradual weight loss, not as fast as some of the "crash" diets we see on social media or read about on the internet. But you will experience a feeling that you will want to feel daily and for the long haul. The sensation of knowing your body is in its optimal healing state is remarkable and is one you will surely look forward to repeating.

Additionally, you will have the added benefit of being sure to savor your next meal. The joy of breaking an extended fast will become a sheer pleasure resulting in a heightened eating experience. You will also be able to enjoy more acutely the flavors at your very next meal. Smaller portions will become your new normal, and your afternoons will be fueled with increased energy and clarity. Much to your disbelief, your mind will become more and more mentally acute. How do I dare make such claims, you might ask? Because I have the pleasure of experiencing this phenomenon daily. Nearly every word in this book has been written by me while in a ketogenic state. As my late British mate would have raised a glass and cheered with that joy filled smile of his, "Brilliant!"

Beginning September 22, 2022, a couple of buddies and I set out on a five-day adventure motorcycle trip. Our trip would start in Colorado, continue into Utah, clip the corner of Wyoming, and conclude crossing the Idaho/Utah state line. We would begin by towing our bikes for the first 225 miles, ride our motorcycles the next 450 miles, and return home towing our bikes the final 245 miles. It would be a total round trip of just over 900 miles. Our plan was to complete the last two stages of the six-stage Utah Backcountry Discovery route (see the Utah route at ridebdr. com). The Utah route consists of predominantly dirt roads across the entire state up to the Idaho border. We had already completed the Colorado route a couple of years ago, and we were two-thirds through the Utah route. This year, unlike other years, I was anxious to see if I would be able to complete each stage while riding my motorcycle in an intermittent fasting, ketogenic state.

In previous years, we would start with a hearty *stick to your ribs* type breakfast just like Grandma said we should. We were sure our bodies needed fuel just as our motorcycles needed fuel. Certainly, we would not have the stamina to ride such technical dirt roads without fueling up our bodies. Makes perfect sense. Well … Dr. Mattson is a track and field coach and has been known to run marathons while on one of his daily fasts. Yes, 26.2 miles of running for four hours with *nothing* in his stomach! If he could do that, I could surely ride a motorcycle for four hours while fasting, right?

Mattson writes about a phenomenon that occurred when a study was conducted on the effects of using ketone ester in liquid form during endurance training (ketone ester is beta hydroxybutyrate or BHB). He tells of five Oxford studies done by Kieran Clark and Pete Cox on thirty-nine elite British cyclists. "In all five studies they found that ketone ester improved the performance of the cyclists by providing *their* muscle cells a fuel (BHB) for efficient production of mitochondria. The cyclists taking the ketone ester also had lower levels of lactate in their blood, which is consistent with their ability to go faster and longer without fatiguing" (Mattson 2022, 139). Prior to the year 2012, no British rider had ever won the Tour de France. Since the taking of BHB in liquid form began, a British rider would win six of the next nine Tour victories. The same ketone ester (BHB) is produced in the body during fasting. Just sayin'.

On the morning of September 23, 2022, my buddy, Mike Hawkins, and I got a brief aerobic workout in pushing our friend Brian Wray's bike around the parking lot in an attempt to get his motorcycle running. The battery was shot, so the first order of business was to get everyone's bikes fired up and ready to hit the trail. Forty-five minutes later, Brian was able to get his bike running by jump-starting it with his truck. We set out on the route at about 9:45 a.m. The total length of the day's route was 150 miles, so it was imperative that we make good time given this was the longest of the two days of riding, and we'd gotten a later start than anticipated.

At 1:39 p.m. we stopped to take a break and have a little snack. I ate some of the beef jerky that my wife insisted on packing for me (thanks, Grace); it had become a necessity and was very timely. I was super excited to find I had been in a ketogenic state for just over six and a half hours as I had been fasting for over eighteen and a half hours. Without doubt, my body was performing at its optimal state. I didn't experience any energy loss or fatigue from my ketogenic state. Zero, zilch, nada! Oh, I was hungry all right, but I was able to manage those hunger pangs by staying well hydrated. It was exhilarating! We rode the final forty miles of the day to the Lincoln Highway 30 tavern in Evanston, Wyoming, where Hawkins and I enjoyed a much-needed cold drink and appetizer served up by a somewhat quintessential Wyoming country girl named Ms. Ricky Lee. Brian even found a NAPA auto parts store that carried the replacement battery he needed for his adventure bike, so we wouldn't have a repeat of that morning the next day.

The next morning, we set out bright and early on the final 120 miles of our trip with the goal of finishing at the Idaho border. My previous day's experiment of riding while fasting in a ketogenic state had put me in a rather cheerful mood. As a matter of fact, I was thrilled. Here I was doing what I enjoy doing with a couple of friends who may have been thinking I had a screw or two loose, but I was doing it well and getting all the benefits that God created our bodies to experience. We completed our four-and-a-half-hour ride to the Idaho border, at about 1:00 p.m. My last meal was at seven the previous night, so that meant I had fasted another eighteen hours, and I felt amazing! We pulled into Cooper's restaurant in Fish Haven, Idaho, for a much-needed lunch break. Upon completion, Hawkins headed back since he was informed his daughter had just given birth to a baby boy in Longmont, Colorado. Brian and I would head over to the Bear Lake cabins in St. Charles, Idaho, where we would bunker down before our eight-hour return trip the next morning; all the while I would be on an intermittent fast, of course.

During our five-day trip, I was able to stick to the intermittent fasting eating patterns the entire time. Prior to our adventure trip, I was not sure whether I would be able to endure the four- to five-hour dirt road sections, because of the energy necessary to complete each day's ride. The whole purpose of doing the rides while in a ketogenic state was to see if Mattson's claim of the boosting effects from ketone ester (BHB) was true. And it was! I'd put science to the test and had proven the positive effects of exerting energy while in a ketogenic state was sound.

Now for the last leg home, that's another story altogether. For the reader simply looking to explore the benefits of exerting energy while in a ketogenic state, the final section of this chapter may not be for you. But for those interested in reading a testimony that focuses on how God works out the details in His creation and in His children's lives, this section is worth reading. The adventure was not quite finished yet, and it was so unimaginable that I have to tell you what God did for me. It was remarkable!

The final stage was an eighty-mile trip on the pavement back to our vehicles parked at the top of Daniel's Pass. This would be our final ride before we would load up our machines for the remaining 250 miles to Maverick Meadow Ridge. Maverick Meadow Ridge is a ranch located just outside of Steamboat Springs where we would settle in for the night and watch Russel Wilson and the Denver Broncos take on the San Francisco 49ers on Sunday night football.

At noontime after a seventeen-hour fast, Brian and I stopped and had lunch at Chick's Café in Heber City, Utah. After lunch, we headed up to Daniel's Summit Lodge and quickly loaded up the bikes, to hit the road by 1:00 p.m. That would leave plenty of time to pick up some pizza in Craig on our way to Steamboat to eat while watching our beloved Broncos. I was following Bryan, and we were making great time approaching Craig at about 4:15 when *snap*! I felt a huge tug on the back of the SUV, like what a skydiver might feel when he or she pulls the rip cord followed by a sudden jolt. The back of the vehicle was suddenly four hundred pounds lighter. I looked in the rearview mirror and saw nothing! My bike was gone! I stopped on the road's shoulder as soon as I could (Thank God there was a shoulder) and scurried around to the rear of my vehicle to find that one of the tie-down straps had snapped. The bike had flipped off the rack onto the street, the other strap held firmly, and I had dragged my motorcycle some forty or so yards before stopping on Colorado's State Highway 40.

I immediately called Brian, letting him know what had just happened, and he promptly turned his vehicle around, trailer and all, to circle back and help me. Thankfully, the traffic during that time of day on a state highway was very light. Over the next twenty-five minutes or so, it took everything we had to muscle the bike back onto the rack, strap it down properly, and make our way safely to Steamboat, albeit with a significantly banged-up bike. We were back on track.

As I was driving the last half hour to Maverick Meadow Ridge, I suddenly became filled with overwhelming joy. My new KTM 790 Adventure bike was banged up rather badly, but I didn't care. The Holy Spirit began to reveal to me what had just taken place, and my mind was flooded with memories of what happened just nine days prior. The plan had always been to part ways at Daniels Summit Lodge because we were all heading home in different directions. Brian was heading east, Mike had already left to visit his new grandson, and I was heading south to Castle Rock. I would then make the two-hour trek to Price, Utah, spend the night and head home the next morning fresh for my seven-hour trip down south.

We made these plans and booked the hotels five full months in advance of our trip. All three of us agreed that we had a good plan, and all of us put the details into our calendars. On September 16, Brian sent me an email out of the blue saying, "Instead of you going south to Price, you could follow me home to Steamboat, then head home on Monday. It's a little farther, but less expensive." I thought, what the heck? My trip would be lengthened by three hours on Sunday when I would be tired, but it would be shortened three hours on Monday.

"OK," I replied. "Consider it done." I canceled my stay in Price and planned on following Brian to Steamboat.

As I was driving, I started calculating where my bike would have fallen off if I had stuck to the original plan. Steamboat was a five-hour drive from Daniel's Lodge, and Price was only a drive of two hours. My tie down strap snapped four hours and fifteen minutes into the trip to Steamboat. That means it would have snapped two hours and fifteen minutes the next day after I had left Price, which would place me on the much-traveled Interstate 70 somewhere between Green River, Utah, and the Colorado state line. In other words, it would have snapped in the middle of nowhere without cell service, by myself, with no hope of lifting the 415-pound motorcycle on an interstate loaded with semitrucks and weekend travelers. I would have been in dire straits. But it did not happen! Praise God!

One way to view the day's events is to say, "Wow, you were so lucky that Brian changed his mind at the last minute and asked you to stay at his place. Otherwise, your motorcycle strap would have snapped the following morning two hours into your trip, leaving you stranded in the High Plains!"

Yes, that's one way, but I prefer a different view. God, our Creator, who is outside of time and space, knew I was going to hastily strap my bike down incorrectly, with the strap rubbing against a piece of metal causing it to break, and knew the incident was going to happen at a time and place that would cause me great distress and put me in grave danger. Because He loves me, God the Holy Spirit either sent a guardian angel or did the job Himself by tapping Brian on the shoulder to suggest he should invite me to stay over at his place Sunday night. Either way, on that day, the infinite God stepped into His finely tuned finite creation to care for one of His children. When the strap did eventually break, Brian would be right there with me to help me in a much safer, calmer environment than would have yielded had we stuck to our original plans. I was overwhelmed by joy at this revelation! God's protection was revealed to me that afternoon, and it was not a result of random chance. No, He knew I would be in this position before He even created me. Praise you, Lord for your protection! By the way, the Broncos won by a single point after a last-minute comeback orchestrated by their new superstar quarterback. Joyous, indeed!

Chapter 5

A Body Designed to Heal

Early in the preface of his book, we discovered that Dr. Matson attributed our body's ability to obtain the benefits associated with intermittent fasting as the result of a meticulous "evolutionary sculpting process." He writes, "As you will discover in this book, evolution has _sculpted_ our cells and organ systems such that they respond to intermittent fasting in ways that enable them to function optimally" (Mattson 2022, xi). By this point, hopefully you've discovered this _optimal_ state is truly astonishing. It's something we would have never been able to learn had it not been for the work of Mattson and his colleagues during their years long endeavor into the scientific research on the topic. We are truly fortunate to have his work and grateful he has revealed these amazing truths.

I am neither a scientist nor a doctor, so I have nothing that I would attempt to contribute to his findings. We would do well to let the facts, as presented, speak for themselves. I have come to believe the evidence he put forth in his book, and his motives for doing so are genuine. There appears to be no profit motivation, which is admirable and rare. I witnessed this myself when I discovered and watched a Ted Talk presentation titled "Why fasting bolsters brain power." After studying Mattson's work, it has become clear to me that he has every intention to help others, and his goal is simply to help the general population optimize their health.

I do, however, differ in one area. I differ as to whom, or what, gets the credit for the astonishing facts revealed in his work. The _benefits_ of eating in intermittent fasting patterns and the fact that it optimizes one's overall health is firmly established in his research; this is undisputed.

But the question remains as to how we ended up with these amazingly complex, self-healing bodies that we now get to enjoy. Was it the *purposeful* act of our bodies being created by God in His image, or was it the result of an atheistic evolutionary process that crafted and sculpted our bodies randomly over billions of years?

Chaos in the Garden—Genesis 3:6–7

All my Christian friends stand on the fact that God is our creator. Many believe, as I do, that He created us in a literal six days as written in the book of Genesis. Others believe creation resulted from the process known as theistic evolution. The scientific community has *largely* become tethered to the theory that life sprung from nonlife billions of years ago, and through the process of natural selection—using the death centered survival of the fittest model—evolved randomly into who or what we are today. So which belief is true?

Theistic evolution proclaims *God* created life and all matter needed to support life. Despite the massive improbabilities, the universe appears to have been precisely *tuned* for this life. They claim that God put the evolutionary process into motion. Over time, humans evolved into who we are today (Collins 2006, 199–200). Doctor and scientist Collins, who is himself a Christian, makes his assertion all the while failing to address what we have identified as "the sin problem." When it comes to sin and the accepted evolutionary theory, there is a contradiction with what the Bible says about sin and its effects upon the Earth and upon humanity. We read of this dichotomy in the book of Romans: "For the wages of sin [is] death, but the gift of God [is] eternal life in Christ Jesus our Lord" (Rom. 6:23 NKJV).

Since the wages of sin is death, and because Jesus lived a perfectly sinless life, He was not required to *pay* those wages. He had no sin; therefore, death could not hold him. Thus, when they crucified Him, after three days He rose.

Just as Jesus was sinless, Adam and Eve were sinless up until the point when they disobeyed God and ate from the tree of the knowledge of good and evil. Since sin had yet to enter God's creation, there were no wages to be paid; thus, there was no death. Evolution is dependent on the reality of death, so how could natural selection by survival of the fittest have even taken place since nothing had died? It couldn't. It didn't.

Mischievous little Atheists

Given that our schools, media, culture, and atheists have worked for decades to create a materialistic system that could explain away God by means of science, evolutionists have created a system where life could exist, in its current form, without a creator. Because science has accepted this flawed theory for decades, in response, some believers have adopted a theory known as theistic evolution. Their hands were tied, in a sense, because they believed the Bible was the true, infallible, inerrant Word of God and, to their credit, held to that belief. They believe God is the creator of everything, which stands in direct opposition to the materialistic theory of evolution being pushed by the scientific and academic communities. So many felt the pressure to align their beliefs with the cultural narrative that the scientific community had eagerly embraced.

Theistic evolutionists espouse that God put into place all things necessary for life, and through a *finely tuned* process of evolution, He sculpted that life into what it is today. The only problem being that there is no basis for this theory in scripture, and as we already covered is impossible given the timing when death entered the world. So how did they come up with this idea of evolution in the first place, given the fact that it is not found in the Bible?

It began with the scientific community. They simply took what was widely known as a theory and began to state it as a fact: evolution through survival of the fittest. They saw a void, and they filled it. Just as Tom Sawyer didn't want to work on his aunt's fence while the other kids were out playing and came up with a mischievous plan to get his playmates to do the work *for* him. The evolutionists did the same with the scientific community.

The atheistic evolutionists proceeded to assiduously paint their fence with such careful precision, checking each application with precise exactness at *every* stroke all the while observing their *finest* work yet. And just like all the neighborhood kids, science could not resist the urge to fill the void and paint the fence *for* them. Or if you prefer, the scientific community "took the ball and ran with it."

Scientists were so enamored with the cultivation, conviction, and dedication of the materialistic, atheistic evolutionists' views on a godless evolutionary theory that they simply agreed to call it science. Given the scientific communities obstinate insistence of declaring this well-known theory as fact, it is easy to see how some Bible-believing Christians would eventually come to the same conclusion; hence, theistic evolution. Go figure?

Notwithstanding the shortfalls of theistic evolution, we thank our friends for giving God all the credit and glory for His creation, no matter *how* they believe He may have done it. Quite the opposite is true of the atheistic, materialistic, Darwinian theory of evolution. This theory attempts to eliminate God from the equation entirely. Darwinian evolutionism is less of a theory and more of a materialistic godless religion. A religion that somehow accepts a myth as truth, believing life sprang into existence from nonlife absent a Creator.

Eric Metaxas in his book *Is Atheism Dead* points out what he insightfully sees as two unavoidable questions when it comes to the origin of life. First, how *did* this indescribable variety of life *come* to be? Answer [from materialists]: "Everything happened by accident randomly evolving from a single cell all the way up to life that now exists." Metaxas's second question is even more important. How did the first life on earth come into being out of nonlife?

For the Christian who believes in creation, the answer is easy, "Well, God, of course. He created *all* life."

The answer from Christians who believe in *theistic evolution* is also easy. God of course, for He created life and put the evolutionary process in motion, so that His creation would eventually evolve into what it is today.

For the materialists who believe that matter is the only thing that exists, having latched themselves to Darwinian evolutionism, they *have* no answer; we just got lucky, I guess (Metaxas 2021, 85).

The Bible paints a different picture entirely. Our finely tuned bodies are the result of God creating them ever so meticulously into the very the image of Himself. The extensive benefits of eating in time restricted eating patterns did not come upon us randomly by chance over billions of years.

In Genesis chapter 1 we read, "In the beginning God created the heavens and the earth. The earth was without form, and void; and darkness was on the face of the deep. And the Spirit of God was hovering over the face of the waters" (vv.1–2).

In the beginning (time), God created the heavens (space) and the Earth (matter), and the Spirit of God was hovering (energy) over the face of the Earth. Time, space, matter, and energy were created in the beginning by God: God the Father, God the Son (John 1:1) and God the Spirit. According to the Bible, life did not come from a prebiotic, primordial soup struck by lightning. No. "In Him was life, and the life was the light of men" (John 1:4 NKJV). Life came from God! Period.

The following account is a brief expositional explanation of what took place during the creation week.

Genesis 1:3: God created light. He did so by letting the light that already existed, the Word of John 1:1, the second person of the trinity, shine upon the Earth before He created the sun and the moon on day 4. We know this to be true because Psalm 72:17 declares His name would continue *"as long as"* the sun. The Hebrew word translated "as long as" is the word *panim*. In the original Hebrew text, the word is defined as before and behind. In the Hebrew, the verse reads "His name shall continue before and behind the sun." This verse shows that Jesus provided the light before God created the sun (Tsarfati 2022).

Genesis 1:4: God puts the Earth into rotation separating light from darkness.

Genesis 1:8: God created the atmosphere.

Genesis 1:9: God divided dry land and seas.

Genesis 1:11: God created plant life.

Genesis 1:14: God tilted the Earth's axis, which would create seasons as well as putting the Earth into orbit to create years in anticipation of His next creation.

Genesis 1:16: God created the sun and the moon.

Genesis 1:17: God put the sun and the moon into place.

Genesis 1:20: God created aquatic and bird life according to their kinds.

Genesis 1:24: God created animal life.

Genesis 1:26: God created mankind.

In the book of Genesis, God tells us that He spoke life into existence (Gen. 1:20, 24, 26). His love for His creation is beyond measure. We are not single-celled organisms that randomly evolved into what we are today. Rather, we are an intentional creation of God, and we were fearfully and wonderfully made, not a fortuitous accident. Praise you, Lord (Ps. 139:14).

Many liberal biblical scholars claim the first five books of the Bible, known as the Pentateuch (five books), written by Moses, are not to be taken literally. They are to be taken allegorically. That is, they say it didn't really happen word for word as written. According to the *Oxford Languages Dictionary*, an allegory is a story, poem, or picture that can be interpreted to reveal a hidden meaning, typically a moral or political one. For example, an allegorical interpretation of Adam and Eve would say those two biblical characters are only there to represent *all* males and females, regardless of what *stage of evolution* they were purported to be in. Similarly, the flood, as recorded by Moses, certainly could not have been an actual *dinosaur-killing* flood, which proceeded to deposit its kill in concentrated regions across the globe, creating visible striations such as the ones found in places like the Grand Canyon, because, let's face it, that would be the silly faith of those naïve Christian folk. More readily, liberal scholars would say the flood account simply represents how God saved humankind from destruction by means of a Savior.

While the latter is certainly true and points to the person of Jesus Christ, the former has some serious misgivings. Adam and Eve did exist (Mark 10:6), the flood did happen (Jesus said so, Luke 17:26–27), the flood killed off most of the dinosaurs (sixty different kinds made it through on the ark, Clarey 2015, 22), dinosaur graveyards were washed into concentrated regions during rising floodwaters, and floodwaters carved out the Grand Canyon as the water receded. The lack of erosion between the layers of sediment tells us it did not happen over billions of years but happened quite suddenly. "The rocks don't lie. Fossils do not show any hint of evolution, only sudden appearance, stasis, then disappearance. Only a global flood can bury the same types of fossils in the same approximate order all over the world at the same time as seal level rose higher and higher" (Clarey 2020, 396).

As written, the Bible is literally true. Those who choose to allegorize scripture are making the choice to water down God's word. Not a good choice. When we take the Bible as literal, we are confronted with many issues, like the issue of original sin. If we allow materialists, atheists, and other belief systems to cause us to allegorize scripture attempting to align with their narrative, we are, in a sense, embracing the omission of original sin altogether. This is convenient for nonbelievers, but a dangerous precedent for believers.

The definition of sin is to "miss the mark." God's word tells us how to live and how to enjoy all the benefits for which He created us. Prior to Adam and Eve's missing the mark, there was no sin, thus, there was no death. Romans 6:23 tells us, "The wages of sin is death." That would mean that the absence of sin would result in the absence of death. Thus, according to the Bible, there would be no "natural selection," which could have only happened if there was death. Likewise, there would be no "survival of the fittest," since all life would have survived until after Adam's sin.

'Til Death Do Us Part

> In the beginning, God created the heavens and the earth. (Gen. 1:1 NKJV)

> God said, "Let Us make man in Our image … In the image of God, He created him; male and female He created them" (Gen. 1:26–27 NKJV)

> Because you have eaten from the tree of which I commanded you [not to eat] saying, "you shall not eat of it." Cursed is the ground for your sake; In toil you shall eat of it all the days of your life. Both thorns and thistles it shall bring forth for you, and you shall eat the herb of the fields. In the sweat of your face, you shall eat bread [un]till you return to the ground. For out of it you were taken; For dust you are. And to dust you shall return. (Gen. 3:17–19 NKJV)

God created humankind with free will; that is, He gave us the ability to choose to obey or disobey. Because of the lust of his eyes and desires of his heart, man chose to disobey God. The result was the fall of humankind and the corruption of God's creation. Sin had entered the world, and it did not take long for that sin to envelop *all* of creation. God's creation was now subject to the laws of thermodynamics. The second law of thermodynamics states that everything tends toward randomness and disorder. If life somehow were to miraculously "evolve" from nonlife, this newfound life would tend toward randomness and disorder. This is the exact opposite of natural selection.

According to Dr. Tour, the more time passes, the worse things become. Time is the enemy of abiogenesis, not the Savior (Metaxas 2021). This observable scientific fact is in complete opposition to Darwin's theory of natural selection, and survival of the fittest claims everything was, and still is, evolving. Before Adam there was no evolution, no sin, no death, and no natural selection process.

The first law of thermodynamics defines that energy can be transformed from one form to another but can neither be created nor destroyed; something cannot come from nothing. As the scientific community continues to cling to the idea of abiogenesis (nonlife to life), they are still faced with the contradiction of the second law, which they conveniently ignore. The genetic makeup of sinful man would eventually suffer the effects of sin by being diseased, unhealthy, and experiencing a finite life span, which was not in God's original plan.

As considered earlier, it is worth repeating. Some might question whether God was "caught off guard" by not anticipating that the free will of humankind to choose would result in them sinning, causing a permanent separation from God and His creation. This is by no means the case. God was not at all surprised by Adam's choice. In His foreknowledge, outside the scope of time and space, He knew exactly what humankind was going to do. That's why He predestined a solution before creation. He created us in a way by which we would be able to deal with the problem of sin. He sent a Savior.

Genesis 3:15 is the first mention of a Savior, the seed of the woman, whom God would send to deal with this sin problem. God is a Holy God, and we sinners cannot be in His presence. Because of God's foreknowledge of this eventuality, He predestined that we would be saved by His Son to remedy the problem. Eternity stepped into time and space to save us. But because the wages of sin is death, and Jesus lived a sinless life, death could not hold Him. Thus, Jesus paid the price as the substitutionary atonement for our sin. When God looks upon us in our sinful state, He sees only Christ because we have been clothed in Him just as we have been endued by the Holy Spirit (Luke 24:49).

We see an example of this type of substitutionary atonement recorded a little further along in Genesis. In this instance, we see a ram caught in the thicket where God the Father provided a substitutionary atonement for the life of Isaac. Isaac, the one and only son of the promised seed mentioned in Genesis 3:15, was as good as dead in his father's eyes for three days on their way to the place of the sacrifice. Just as Jesus was sacrificed at the same location some two-thousand years later and where His body lay for three days.

God took care of, once and for all, the spiritual condition that resulted from humankind's sin. But what about our physical condition, you ask? I would submit to you that God had a predetermined solution for that as well. All we need do is follow the eating patterns that He gave us in His Word and taught to His people. Our *finely tuned* bodies will do the rest.

The fact is that God created a perfectly *fine-tuned* universe. He also created a perfectly *fine-tuned* Earth, complete with a tilted axis providing the benefit of having different seasons, of which the rotation on that axis gives us days and nights, a perfect atmosphere to support plant and animal life, and at a precise location enabling the earth to be inhabited with precisely fine-tuned life. Whether it be plant life, animal life, or human life, God created it with intention and without the aid of the made-up theory we call evolution.

Give It a Rest

A fascinating example of restoration can be observed in one of God's commandments. His people were to let the ground lay fallow for a time after every sixth year of harvest, so the land could restore itself. God even gave us an example of this kind of rest after His six days of creation when He did as such for one day. As we can now see, God had a similar plan for our bodies. We are to let our stomachs *lay fallow, or rest, daily.* He Created the Earth to rest for 14.3 percent of a seven-year period, and He created our bodies to be in a ketogenic state for at least 14.3 percent, or 3½ hours each day. Coincidence?

Here in the United States of America, we have essentially had the luxury of eating large breakfasts followed by lunch, then capped off with a well-portioned dinner often including dessert or a light snack before bed. In the nineteenth century, our medical community's established practices believed that the body being adequately stuffed with food was necessary for strength, vitality, and a cure-all for what ails you. They thought it was of great importance to keep food in their stomachs, at all times, in order to obtain optimal health. No breaks, no fasts, and no time to let the stomach rest or "lay fallow." They even used what we now know as barbaric practices such as forced feedings of predigested foods and daily whiskey and milk regimens, ensuring these practices were administered twenty-four hours a day, seven days a week, at all cost. The goal was to reduce sickness and fever and promote good health whether the patient had the constitution to endure such practices or not. Usually not. Death frequently ensued (Dewey 1894).

We now know that filling our stomachs in perpetuity does not promote good health; rather, being in this state has proven contrary to the metabolic health that is necessary to optimize overall results. Knowing that humankind would end up in a fallen state, God sculpted our cells and organs so they would be able to *adapt* to this new condition. In previous chapters, we saw how God demonstrated His care for His creation by teaching them to eat in time-restricted eating patterns, so they could take full advantage of *their finely* tuned bodies.

Because of the work that Dr. Mark Mattson performed over his thirty-plus-year career at Johns Hopkins University, we now see a clear picture of how our perfectly *sculpted* organisms enable us to cope with illnesses such as obesity, aging, disease prevention, cardiovascular disease, stroke, type 2 diabetes, Alzheimer's and Parkinson's diseases, as well as improved brain synapses and neural network activity.

In the beginning, God created the heavens and the Earth. Subsequently, Satan and his angels fell as a result of Satan's hubris desire to be like God. The earth was formless and void, at which point God the Father, God the Son, and God the Spirit (Gen. 1:2; John 1:1–3, 14) began the creation process by which They created our Earth in a literal six twenty-four-hour periods. Upon the completion of this process, God saw that it was indeed good. (Gen. 1:3–31) God was in no way surprised by Satan's rebellion and the fall of humankind. In His foreknowledge, He knew His creation would become subject to the effects of sin, so He predetermined the solution, because He loves us. For God so loved *His Creation* that He gave His only begotten Son, that whoever believes in Him *as savior* should not perish but have everlasting life. (John 3:16) God was not and never will be either surprised or caught off guard. From the beginning He had a solution to save our souls *and* to allow our physical bodies to thrive as well.

Chapter 6

Meal Planning

You Are ~~What~~ *When* You Eat

What if I told you that *when* you eat is more important than *what* you eat. The matter of when you eat becomes a question of whether you prefer burning carbs as your energy source or burning fat. We are going to see how God created our bodies to burn fat while at the same time resulting in extensive additional health benefits. In the spring of 2021, Grace and I decided to take on what is known as the Talon's challenge in the middle of the upcoming ski season. The Talon's challenge is a snow skiing event created to benefit youth sports in Eagle County, Colorado. The 2022 season would be the nineteenth running of the annual event, and it would once again be held on the Birds of Prey runs at Beaver Creek Resort. The Challenge was to ski 26,226 vertical feet consisting of fourteen black and double black diamond ungroomed mogul bump runs in one day. The event would begin at 9:00 a.m., with the last chair closing at 3:30 p.m. Yikes! Quite the challenge.

As far as Grace's ability to complete this challenge, no problem. She would even do it on her snowboard, which is rarely attempted at this event. As for me, that was a different story. I was way too out of shape. I had already skied each of the runs in the past year but certainly not in one day. I was well aware of the task at hand, and I understood that in my current condition I would have no chance. Even worse, I told everyone I knew that I was going to be taking on this challenge, so there was no backing out. I figured the peer pressure would motivate me to get into Double Black

Diamond ski condition, and it did. Because I was now fully committed to taking on this challenge, I did two things. First, I started a daily workout regimen, and second, I started counting my calories; I needed to drop some serious weight.

On February 26, 2022, Grace and I were ready to go. I had exercised pretty consistently during the past nine months; my legs and back were considerably stronger, and my cardiovascular system was much improved (you get really winded when skiing moguls at altitude). By the afternoon of the event, Grace and I were on the brink of completing the challenge. We rode the last chair up the mountain at 2:00 p.m., and we finished at 2:30 p.m., one hour before the chairlifts were to close.

We did it. Yes! It must have been a piece of cake given that we finished an hour early, right? Not a chance, not for me, anyway. I had only lost about five pounds prior to the event, and my goal was to lose much more. I tried to do it by exercising and cutting calories, but for me I found doing this consistently was quite difficult and frustrating. I would preplan meals; I downloaded calorie-counting apps; I tried to stop eating anything that would put me above my daily caloric intake goals. You name it, I tried it. All good things for sure, but for me it was sort of a bummer. I always enjoyed a good meal and delighted in that piece of banana cream pie, but not any longer. No sir! I had a mountain to conquer!

A couple of weeks prior to taking on the Talon's Challenge, I started eating in one of the intermittent fasting patterns that Mattson outlined in his newly released book. I began by committing to a 16/8 pattern. I even skipped breakfast and did not eat until 10:00 a.m. the day of the event. I would typically finish my last meal of the day around 7:00 p.m. and fast until about 11:00 a.m. the following day. After a few weeks, I was able to work my way up to a 17/7 pattern. The results were miraculous. Over the next six months, I lost about ten pounds, and I wasn't even dieting! Inches were coming off my waist, and people started noticing. "Hey, you're looking pretty good. Is that a new shirt?"

"As a matter of fact, it is. Let me tell you about my new eating pattern." All I needed to do was eat in the prescribed eating pattern that I had recently discovered. I was enjoying much greater freedom with my food choices, and I was feeling grrrrreat—every day even without the Frosted Flakes. I had transitioned from burning carbs in the mornings as my energy source to burning fat from the ketones my body would create. The daily twelve-hour fast would trigger my body to flip its metabolic switch, and all I needed to do was remain in that optimal state for an additional three to five hours daily.

Now, to be sure, I was very careful with the liberty that I had discovered with this newly adopted eating pattern. When consumed at the correct time, good food is always good for you, and whether consumed at the correct time or not, bad food is always bad for you. Nonetheless, with the freedom that comes from eating after a fast, my definition of good and bad was changing. If you will forgive me, it was *evolving*, in a metaphorical sense, of course. As the saying goes, *everything in moderation* for sure. But then again, I no longer thought of that slice of pie after dinner as *bad*; rather, I found that eating it after 7:00 p.m. was the issue. Additionally, no longer did I view having an In-N-Out burger as harmful; rather, I would have it with a zero-calorie drink, skip the fries, and only have the burger to break my fast around the noontime hour.

As the weeks and months of eating in time-restricted eating patterns went by, I found I also *wanted* to eat healthier. The knowledge that my body was benefiting from letting my stomach lay fallow for a full twelve hours made me not want to put bad things into it. I felt amazing, and the last thing I wanted to do was fill my stomach with some sort of gut bomb and ruin the incredible benefits I was experiencing. Even at this very moment, it is 12:35 p.m. on a Saturday, and I refuse to eat until I finish this section. If I do, that *rich blood* Dewey spoke of will leave my brain to attend to my stomach.

I found myself naturally desiring healthier options such as entrée salads, tuna and crackers, a deli sandwich, or maybe some leftovers from the previous evening's meal. Because I would always stay well hydrated, I was not famished or starved as the lunch hour approached as some might think. As a matter of fact, if I was locked in and busy with the task before me, I hardly even noticed.

Another funny thing started happening; I found that I was enjoying my lunchtime meals more than ever. I was tasting every single ingredient, savoring them like never before. And funnier yet, I found I was eating less. No more did I binge on those waffle fries; the grilled chicken sandwich was enough; just not on Sundays, if you hear what I'm sayin'. The fruit cup sounded better and better, and the entrée salads (meat included) were tasting incredible. I tried to consistently finish my last meal of the day by 7:00 p.m., but I didn't always accomplish that goal. It didn't matter. I would still fast after dinner until around noon the next day. Smaller servings were beginning to be preferred over larger ones.

My stomach was shrinking and the fat surrounding it had begun to dissipate. I came to really enjoy the feeling of having a tasty meal and not feeling stuffed afterward. I even began to enjoy having a midmorning empty stomach. It energized me mentally because I knew my body had flipped the metabolic switch, and I was reaping the benefits of being in a ketogenic state. That is, my body was creating all the good stuff that God created it to make. I was getting healthier at that very moment, and my growling stomach was a constant reminder of how good I felt, and of how good God is for creating me this way.

Tips Included

It may not be a full 20 percent, but I feel the need to tip you anyway. The following are a few tips to remember as you begin your intermittent fasting journey.

When you wake up in the morning, drink water—*lots* of water. It will rehydrate you from the night's rest and help sustain you until you are ready to break your fast around lunchtime. If you enjoy a soft drink, make sure it does not have sugar. Drink your coffee black with no creamer (the intake of cream, which contains energy, will break your fast), and if you prefer sweetener in your coffee or tea, make sure it is an artificial sweetener containing no calories such as monk fruit or stevia. Coffee is also an appetite suppressant, so that may help you as well. Stay away from Starbucks until you break your fast. (I would say, stay away from Starbucks, period. Just think how much money you will save?!)

If you find you cannot have that morning coffee without a dash of milk, cream, or sweetener, no worries. Just try to keep the caloric intake to a minimum. One of the people I work with told me she was going to commit to a 15/9 intermittent fasting eating pattern for the next two weeks. She planned to stop eating at 8:00 p.m. and would not eat again until 11:00 a.m. the following day. Two weeks later she was happy to report she had lost five pounds without exercise or dieting (exercise was planned to start after the holidays). Four weeks into her journey, she now finishes her evening meals at 8:00 p.m., limits her morning caloric intake, and starts eating her next meal at around 1:00 p.m. that following day. The results are she is feeling fantastic, looking fabulous, and as she will admit, her clothes are getting a little baggy. Good for her!

"I do have to admit," she said, "I have been cheating in the mornings by putting milk in my coffee. I feel guilty."

Don't feel guilty! This is fantastic news! You put yourself into a ketogenic state during your twelve-hour fast by burning the 400 to 500 calories stored in your liver; you broke your fast with 30 to 40 calories of milk and reentered the ketogenic state after quickly shedding within minutes the light caloric intake. You can easily get back into the optimal state that God created for you to be in. Just don't eat breakfast! It's that simple.

When it comes to meals, fresh food is always better. Deep-fried food is never a good idea. Get the grilled chicken sandwich not the fried crispy one; your taste buds will learn to savor it, and you won't need a nap afterward. Choose brioche buns over those big doughy monstrosities; they are much lighter, include far fewer carbs, and are just plain yummy.

Be sure to include ample amounts of fish and chicken in your meals. Fish oils are an excellent source of the good fats, such as Omega-3, that your body needs, and chicken is low in calories, is filled with proteins, and is very versatile. I suggest you not rationalize your healthy choice to eat fish and chicken as you run to the deep-fried fish and chips or the crispy chicken tenders. Those deep-fried meals are tempting and tasty, but they are unhealthy and are sure to put you in a food coma afterward. It's just not worth it. I'm talking about grilled, sautéed, blackened, or broiled chicken or fish. You will feel healthy and vibrant because your body will be using the food for energy, rather than taxing your body by forcing it to digest what it need not digest.

If you want a big juicy steak, go for it! Try using a dry rub for seasoning and stay away from the steak sauce. As you are enjoying dinner, be sure to pay close attention to how you are feeling. You may want to save some of that delicious cut of beef, so you can break your fast with it the following day around lunchtime.

If you haven't figured it out by now, I am not a nutritionist, nor would I ever claim to be one. However, if you suffer from type I diabetes, I recommend you speak to your physician *before* you consider adopting an intermittent fasting pattern. (I would also encourage you to refer to Mattson's book if you have other specific health concerns.)

As mentioned, I'm not a nutritionist rather a businessman with an MBA from the University of Colorado at Colorado Springs. What has recently been revealed to me is that our bodies have been designed so flawlessly that we can thoroughly enjoy eating food. I, as much as anyone, like having a good meal with family, friends, and coworkers. I also love that by employing one of the intermittent fasting patterns as described by Dr. Mattson, I can eat just about anything, and so can you! God designed us that way. He wants us to take pleasure in all His creation. That includes consuming fruits, vegetables, meats, grains, legumes, dairy— all of it!

I began this chapter by telling you how I struggled with counting calories, even when faced with what I saw as an overwhelming physical challenge. I had every motivation to drop my caloric intake and lose the necessary pounds in order to accomplish my upcoming challenge. Much like the motivation the scientific community has had over the past seventy-years with their struggle to re-create the Miller-Urey soup experiment, but I digress. While it is true that burning more calories than one consumes will help someone lose weight, the fact is that it is hard to do, and it can prove detrimental to many if not done in a healthy manner. Just take a look around; it appears to be extremely hard.

Thankfully, God gave us another way to accomplish the goal of optimizing health. He gave us an eating pattern by which our bodies are able to flip the metabolic switch, create ketones from fat cells, and accomplish long-term and sustainable health benefits. All we need to do is follow the time-restricted eating patterns as demonstrated in the Bible, and eat of the healthy, fresh, and delicious bounty that He created for us. Do this in moderate proportions within specific eating windows, and Voila! You are sure to optimize your health and enhance your overall physical performance.

Chapter 7

The Mystery of Exercise Revealed

Here's the deal. Just as this eating pattern is not a diet, it is not an exercise program either. The only thing that is required for you to obtain the benefits of intermittent fasting is that you put your body into a ketogenic state on a regular basis whenever possible. That is, consume *zero* energy intake for a minimum of twelve hours after your last meal. Just stop eating! Every minute after your body consumes the 400 to 500 calories of glucose stored in your liver, you gain the benefits of creating ketones by which your body fuels itself. My personal goal is to go seventeen hours before I break my fast and get to my eating window, but fifteen- and sixteen-hour fasts will benefit you as well, just for a shorter period of time.

Even though this eating pattern is not an exercise program, there is a way to incorporate exercise into your intermittent fasting lifestyle, which will greatly benefit your body and brain. If you stop eating at 6:30 p.m., then at 6:30 a.m. you will be in a ketogenic state. Just as there is an eating window when you adopt the intermittent fasting eating pattern, there is also an exercise window if you want to get the most bang for your buck when fasting. Mattson points out these benefits rise at an accelerated rate when one chooses to add exercise into the equation (Mattson 2022, 103).

My wife and I are members of the United States Olympic and Paralympic Museum in Colorado Springs, but we are certainly *not* Olympic athletes. We are members to support what they stand for, not to be like them. I say this to emphasize you don't need to train like an Olympian either—just up your heart rate a little while in a ketogenic state. You need not train like an Olympic athlete, but your body will reward you as if you did.

Here is my routine. I try to stop eating around 7:00 p.m. I start my short workout around seven the next morning Monday through Friday. That means I am working out in a ketogenic state around twenty to thirty-five minutes four to five times a week. That's it. If that doesn't work in your schedule, try abstaining from eating anytime in the evening, resisting the urge to eat until at least fifteen hours later. Even a short fifteen-minute workout will benefit you because you will have flipped the metabolic switch after the twelfth hour.

After twelve hours of fasting, the glucose in your liver is depleted, stimulating the production of ketones necessary to sustain exercise. Ketones have been found to be much more efficient at sustaining increased activity than glucose. This increase in ketone production bolsters the brain activity and enhances the body's ability to resist stress, injury, and disease (Mattson 2022, 6). Because of the stress placed upon the body after you have flipped the metabolic switch, the body turns on antioxidant genes to reduce free radicals and stimulate the increase of healthy mitochondria, which will enable the cells to become stronger from the stress induced upon it by exercise (Mattson 2022, 48).

He goes on to say three things that need to be done consistently will allow your body to improve its ability to enhance, repair, and protect its DNA. "The take-home message is clear—exercise your neurons, exercise your body and fast intermittently" (Mattson 2022, 51). If we take the doctor's advice to stimulate our brains daily by means of reading, studying, or creating, coupled with frequent exercise, we are sure to see the empirical evidence of improvements to our mental and physical health, and we will be positioned to sustain this healthier lifestyle for the rest of our lives.

If you're needing some exercise inspiration or you simply don't have time to commit to going to the gym, here are some simple activities that will boost ketone production when you are in a ketogenic state. It is simple; do these once your body has eliminated the glucose that was stored in your liver during the past twelve hours, and the ketones created from fat will be used to sustain increased activity. The following are just a few examples of possible activities:

- Take a walk with you dog.
- Do lunges, squats, sit-ups or cordless jump ropes.

- Walk on a treadmill.
- Stream a workout routine app from your phone to your television.
- Jog, run, or ride a bicycle.
- Go up and down stairs.
- Do weight training or aerobic exercise.

You know what activities you enjoy doing the most, so just try doing them while in a ketogenic state. Your energy levels will be at their peak, and you will experience enhanced performance in all that you undertake. I used to make sure I had a full stomach before I would ride my dirt bike or go snow skiing. But I have learned that exercising while fasting puts my energy levels at their peak and my abilities are enhanced more than ever. I perform much better than I did when I had a meal digesting in my stomach, and I feel stronger and more invigorated. I no longer eat before physical activity. I make sure I am well hydrated, and go for it. I encourage you to do the same. If you accept this challenge, I assure you that you are going to find you will outperform what you have done in the past.

Remember, it's not the intensity of the workout that boosts ketone production; rather, it is the fact that your body has flipped the metabolic switch. It has already used all the glucose that was stored in your liver. Now it produces and uses ketones as its energy source. *Any* increase in your heartrate after twelve hours of zero energy input (calories) will result in the extensive health benefits as outlined earlier. Just how God planned it. Praise God!

If you are faced with choosing between exercising in a ketogenic state or spending time with the Lord in devotion and prayer, choose the latter. You will still reap the health benefits because you are following the time-restricted eating pattern as demonstrated in the Bible. How great is that? First come to the Lord spiritually, rest in Him, and let your finely tuned body do the rest. Seek God's kingdom first and all your needs will be added to you (Matt. 6:33). He created us to love Him. He will take care of the rest because *He loves us.*

Chapter 8

Revelations

The following quote was taken from the great murder mystery novelist Agatha Christie. *"The impossible could not have happened, therefore the impossible must be possible in spite of appearances."*

Here we see how Inspector Poirot witnessed something that, given the evidence, appeared to be impossible. As it turned out, the impossible was in fact possible despite its appearance. The Bible is filled with these types of mysteries that, on the surface, appear an impossibility. However, with some study and insight, we discover that they are indeed possible.

The title track to the band NEEDTOBREATHE's album, *Into the Mystery,* begins with the following lyrics: "It's hard to *see* it, [and] still *believe* it. You have *always* lived deep inside my heart." God living inside our hearts? That indeed is a mystery that seems impossible to see and believe. How could the magnificent Creator of the universe live inside me? The reality is the second person of the trinity, the angel of the LORD who spoke to the prophets, is exactly who lives inside you if you will allow Him (John 17:26b). This phenomenon seems impossible until you witness the changes in a person's life who has encountered the living God. You cannot see God, but you can definitely see how He changes people. Some He changes so drastically that your belief in Him is sure to increase. We find these *hard to believe* miracles in many places throughout scripture. One such mystery is found in the Gospel of Mark. Let's examine how this and *other* mysteries of God spoken to us by Jesus strengthen our faith in Him and reveal His goodness toward us, His people.

The Mystery of the Unpardonable Sin

> And He said to them, "To you it has been given to know
> the mystery of the kingdom of God; but to those who are
> [on the] outside, all things come in parables." (Mark 4:11
> NKJV)

Jesus spoke many things during His time on earth. Early on in His ministry, He spoke very clearly and directly to large groups of people. In Matthew chapters five through seven, we find the famous Sermon on the Mount where He spoke to many and taught the beatitudes. Those words were spoken very clearly to the multitudes that gathered on the hillside, and they understood precisely what He was saying. A bit later in His ministry, there came a time when He would not speak to the people so clearly. Rather He would speak to them only in parables, and He would explain those parables privately and exclusively to those closest to Him: His disciples.

What caused the change? The leadership of Israel began committing what the Bible refers to as the *unpardonable sin,* as documented in the Gospel of Matthew. As they heard the lies from the Jewish leadership, the multitudes began to turn on Jesus.

"Therefore, I say to you, every sin and blasphemy will be forgiven men, but the blasphemy [against] the Spirit will not be forgiven men" (Matt. 12:31 NKJV).

So, what is the mystery of the unpardonable sin anyway—a sin that Jesus said is so bad, that the Father in heaven will not even consider forgiving it? It's the only one of its kind. The big question is: have I already committed this sin? Will I? Am I at risk? I mean, Lord knows I have done some pretty sketchy things over the years, some of them pretty bad!

Relax. If you have accepted Jesus as your Lord and Savior, then you have not, cannot, and will not, commit the unpardonable sin. It's too late, you have already been saved—forever. You did nothing to earn salvation, and you can do nothing to lose it either. You might say, "Well, I rejected the Holy Spirit up until the age of forty. Does that mean that I am doomed?" *No,* there is a difference between forgiveness and a pardon. You have already been forgiven; you have yet to be pardoned because you have yet to be judged. When we die, we go to the judgment seat of God. If you accepted Christ as Lord when you were alive, you will immediately be pardoned. If you did not, it's too late. You are guilty! As the soup Nazi once said, *no soup for you! (Seinfeld).*

The unpardonable sin in the Bible is the sin of rejecting the Holy Spirit's message that Jesus is the Messiah. If you listened to the Spirit and accepted the gift of Jesus as your Savior, you are covered—for all eternity.

Dr. Arnold Fruchtenbaum, in his commentary on the life of the Messiah, adds that the unpardonable sin of rejecting Jesus Christ as Messiah was committed by the Jewish nation at the beginning of the common era. The time when Messiah came to earth.

They paid the ultimate price in AD 70 when Rome destroyed Jerusalem and the temple resulting in the Jewish nation being scattered to the ends of the earth.

When it became clear that the Jewish leadership was going to reject Him as their Messiah, Jesus would only reveal His parables regarding the *mystery* of the kingdom of God privately to his closest disciples.

The Mystery of Predestination

"He chose us in Him before the foundation of the world, that we should be holy and without blame before Him in love, having predestined us to adoption as sons by Jesus Christ to Himself, according to the good pleasure of His will" (Eph. 1:4–5 NKJV).

Before the foundation of the world, God ordained those of us who are in Him to be holy and blameless. But He gave us free will and left the matter of whether we would make that choice up to us. Once we exercise our free will and make the choice to be His children, He predestined the results.

Because God is outside of time and is omniscient (all-knowing), He knew who would accept Christ and who would not, even before the foundation of the world. He did not predestine our salvation; rather, he predestined the results of what would happen to us after we chose to accept His Son and become saved. Further down in verse 11 of Eph. 1, we read that once we choose Him, He has predetermined our inheritance, and He has a purpose for us. All we must do is choose to accept His free gift. A gift is only a gift if we choose to accept it.

The Mystery of God

"But in the days of the sounding of the seventh angel, when he is about to sound, the mystery of God would be finished, as He declared to His servants the prophets" (Rev. 10:7 NKJV).

This verse is a prophetic verse penned by the apostle John describing events that will take place in the second half of the tribulation. So, what is the mystery of God that will be finished during the last days? As declared through His servants and prophets through His Word (the Bible) from Genesis 1:1 through Revelation 22:20, the mystery of God that will be declared to all creation in the last days is as follows:

> That God, the creator of the heavens and the Earth, loved us so much, that He sent His one and only Son to die for us as a substitutionary atonement for our sin. This atonement has the power to make us righteous in His eyes, enabling us sinners to be made perfect and be in the presence of a perfect and Holy God for all eternity. He also gave us His Spirit to bear witness of our Savior, Jesus Christ. All we need to do is hear His voice and accept His offer (Tsarfati 2022).

There you have it. Now you *know* it. Run with it. You can no longer say you never knew. Sorry, not sorry.

The Mystery of Good Health

These are just a few of the mysteries of God we can discover when we spend time in His Word. And just as the Mystery of God can be summed up in a couple of short sentences that include unconditionally essential information, so also can summarizing the findings on the mystery of good health be summarized with such ease. Simply adopt an eating pattern where you stop eating at a specific time after your main meal, abstain from snacking after that time, and refrain from eating until around the lunch hour the following day. Take up a daily fast that lasts fifteen to seventeen hours.

This mystery was once revealed in the nineteenth century, but it struggled to become accepted in the twentieth and twenty-first centuries. The dismissal of these ideas came about because of two factors:

1. The lack of high-tech laboratories where one could conduct and document repeatable scientific evidence to back up the resulting benefits.
2. The scientific community's willingness to accept the atheistic theory of Darwinian evolution as fact in an attempt to explain away our existence absent a creator.

Science has now proven that intermittent fasting results in increased overall health, and Eric Metaxas and others have exposed Darwinian evolutionism for what it is: a fraud. But let's take a deeper look into the two factors that have prevented intermittent fasting from really taking hold.

Empirical Evidence

In 1902, Edward Hooker Dewey published *The True Science of Living*. In his book, he went into detail as to how his patients responded positively after exhorting them to skip meals during times of disease and sickness. The results were no less than astounding. In nearly every case, Dr. Dewey witnessed his patients' conditions improving rather than declining as a result of his prescribed methods. Much to the chagrin of the medical establishment of the day, Dr. Dewey discovered the body would, given the right amount of time and circumstance, heal itself when left to its own means. Over the years, he collected as much empirical evidence as one would need in order to make a strong case to adopt this eating pattern. So why was his time-restricted eating pattern rejected? Why were his methods not adopted? The reason Dewey's research was rejected resulted from the answer to a single question. Likewise, Mattson's findings on the topic are being largely ignored because of the answer to that same question.

What Is the Answer to Ninety-Nine out of One Hundred Questions?

To quote a line from David Aames in the movie *Vanilla Sky*, the answer is money! There is big money in the pharmaceutical industry with its current and ever-increasing cash flow. The medical field had every incentive to not let Dewey's findings get out to the general public. The pharmaceutical industry naturally resisted any claim that would champion the idea our bodies are able to heal themselves, without drugs no less and with a treatment that is so simple. It became necessary for them to dismiss Dr. Dewey's findings as heresy invented by a dangerous lunatic (Dewey 1894, 160).

By joining with the established medical professionals that already existed in the medical community, the self-enlightened lemmings marched dutifully over the edge of the cliff, nullifying the gains of any published cure that did not profit them—even if the results included an overwhelming amount of empirical and repeatable scientific evidence. Unfortunately, in Dr. Dewey's case there was little, if any, clinical scientific evidence available at the time to back up his findings. He practiced in the nineteenth century. The technology was just not there—yet.

"In the course of time, as there was a constant addition to the ranks of believers, so the pressure came upon me for a solution of the question which would satisfy the science behind it, if any were to be found, and all the more as my professional brethren were beginning to comment." One went so far as to admit privately that Dewey must be out of his mind for suggesting his patients go without breakfast. "My comfort was, during those earlier times, that all opposition, no matter how couched in ridicule or sarcasm; no matter whether from a professional or a *layman*, was aimed, not at me, but at a larger compliance with the immutable laws of life itself, and hence I could bide my time and did not allow my mind to become soured by opposition, no matter how intense or in what form it came" (Dr. Edward Dewey, ibid.).

Dewey was perpetually challenged on the science behind his findings. It had yet to exist in his era; he was ahead of his time. Yet the medical and pharmaceutical establishments acted quickly and eliminated the threat altogether. Problem solved.

An Observable and Repeatable Scientific Method

In February of 2022, Johns Hopkins University Professor Dr. Mark P. Mattson published his book, revealing his decades-long research on the benefits of using time-restricted eating patterns: *The Intermittent Fasting Revolution.* Dr. Mattson goes into detail revealing how the body can heal itself given the right amount of time and circumstances—just like Dewey witnessed in the nineteenth century. If people would simply change their eating pattern to restrict their eating into a specified window each day and abstain from eating for a period of fifteen to seventeen hours on a consistent basis, in the vast majority of cases, our bodies would heal themselves by their own means.

So why then is Dr. Mattson's research not being widely accepted and applied? For the very same reason Dr. Dewey's findings were rejected; the pharmaceutical industry is big business and even bigger money. They do not want the concept of a self-healing body to take hold with the general public. They have gigantic marketing budgets giving them the ability to own the messaging while suppressing the science. Additionally, they visit doctors' offices and give them free samples to use on their patients, resulting in many doctors prescribing their product whether it's necessary or not. This might sound harmless save the fact that patients have been conditioned for years that popping a pill or taking a poke is sure to cure all ills. Ahhh, I feel better now. Really? Do you?

All that the pharmaceutical industry need do is convince the medical practice to continue their current prescription methods. Or better yet, increase them. After all, healing without medication is simply not possible. Once again, the lemmings march dutifully over the edge of the cliff nullifying the gains of any revealed cure that doesn't involve them— or even worse, anything that might be at risk of lowering their stock valuation. Cynical, yes, but unfortunately, true.

Occam's Razor

There is a second reason why the adoption of restricted eating patterns has not been widely accepted despite the many well-documented health benefits. Of the two doctors we have been referencing, this reason applies only to Mattson's research. The reason is because of something science refers to as Occam's razor. You might ask, what the heck is an Occam's razor? I've heard of Gillette but never Occam. Webster's defines Occam's razor as "a scientific and philosophical rule that entities should not be multiplied unnecessarily which is interpreted as requiring that the simplest of competing theories be preferred to the more complex or that explanations of unknown phenomena be sought first in terms of known quantities." The more complex the answer, the less likely it is correct. In other words, keep it simple.

According to the figure below taken from *The Intermittent Fasting Revolution* found on page 103, Occam's razor would classify the idea of evolutionary sculpting as a nonstarter. Illustration #2

<u>Sculpted by Evolution</u>   or   <u>Created by God</u>

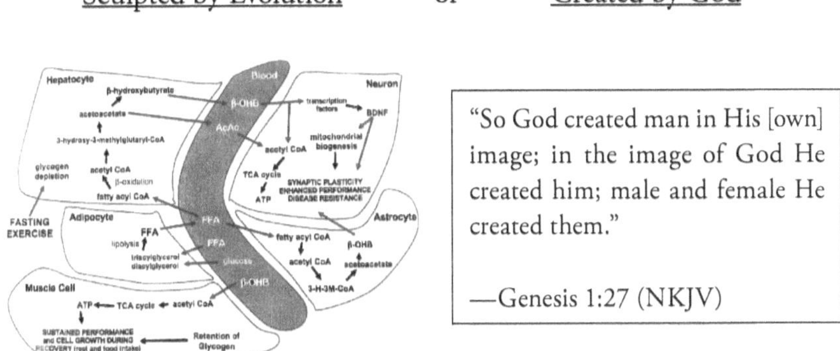

"So God created man in His [own] image; in the image of God He created him; male and female He created them."

—Genesis 1:27 (NKJV)

Mattson's Figure 4.1

During fasting, liver glucose stores (glycogen) are depleted, and blood glucose levels remain low. Next, free fatty acids (FFA) are released into the blood from fat cells. The FFA are then transported into liver cells and converted to the ketones acetoacetate and beta-hydroxybutyrate (BHB). Blood ketone levels rise, and the ketones are transported into cells throughout the body and brain, where they are metabolized to acetyl coenzyme A (CoA), which is then used to produce adenosine triphosphate (ATP). The author's laboratory found that BHB can also stimulate the production of brain-derived neurotrophic factor (BDNF) in neurons.

BDNF facilitates learning and memory and protects neurons against stress. Additional benefits of fasting for cells in the brain, heart, and skeletal muscle are the stimulation of mitochondrial biogenesis and autophagy, which effectively remove damaged molecules and increase the number of healthy mitochondria in the cells. TCA = tricarboxylic acid; OHB = hydroxybutyrate
(Mattson, Mark P. *The Intermittent Fasting Revolution*, 103. MIT Press. Kindle Edition).

The assumption that evolution sculpted us to such a degree of complexity absent a creator is not at all simple. (In fact, it's the opposite of simple.) It is tough for anyone to grasp everything that must take place for this remote evolutionary process to ever have happened.

The idea that *God* sculpted our bodies rather than Darwinian evolution doing the sculpting is gaining more and more appeal as science uncovers more of this mystery. Mattson uncovered an incredible amount of detail of what takes place during an intermittent fasting ketogenic state. We can safely say that the creation model has far fewer assumptions than the evolutionary sculpting theory when we consider the amount of evolution necessary to accomplish the level of detail discovered by the doctor.

So why has this eating pattern struggled to reach the mainstream? Both Dewey's and Mattson's challenge was to overcome the fact that the medical and pharmaceutical industries had and have the money and motivation necessary to ensure their ideas would not take hold despite being proven scientifically. Mattson's additional challenge is selling the idea that our miraculous bodies resulted from a very long, drawn out, meticulously detailed, and seemingly improbable chance evolutionary process. When the truth is laid out, most rational people don't buy it. It's just that simple.

A Light in a Dark World

> Jesus, when teaching his disciples on the mountainside
> said the following: "You are the light of the world. A city
> that is set on a hill cannot be hidden. Nor do they light a
> lamp and put it under a basket, but on a lampstand, and

it gives light to all [who are] in the house. Let your light so shine before men, that they may see your good works and glorify your Father in heaven." (Matt. 5:14–16 NKJV)

Through the work of a brave doctor during the era of the American Civil War and the work of a brilliant university neuroscientist of the twenty-first century, God has revealed to us an eating pattern that optimizes health and enhances performance. These two doctors have revealed a pattern that we also see demonstrated in the Bible. A mystery has been explained.

This revelation has uncovered something that could have a profoundly positive impact on many people around the world if it were to be widely adopted. Dr. Dewey tried to no avail in the nineteenth century; Dr. Mattson has put out a masterful work in the twenty-first century that precisely follows the scientific method, but it has yet to take hold for reasons previously discussed. The question is who can get this eating pattern out to the public? Who can make it stick?

I believe it's the church, that's who! The church can rally around this concept and show the world the positive impact that it can have. Most in the medical community are certainly not going to do so. They have already shown they're so entrenched in their medical practices that anything outside their established norms will quickly be dismissed and/or labeled as nonsensical. Neither will it be the pharmaceutical industry. With the cash flow that has already been injected so intravenously, the very thought of them weaning themselves off that drug might possibly trigger the onset of serious withdrawals.

What about science you ask? Science has advanced to such a point that we can clearly see the health benefits of eating in such patterns. But they have become wedded to materialistic, atheistic, Darwinian evolution. Not a chance they will break up that marriage. The price to pay is just way too high, so they will continue to stay married and learn to live with it.

The reality is that God has used these two men over many years along with His word to reveal another mystery: the mystery of good health. The mystery of an eating pattern that will surely help nearly everyone obtain a healthier lifestyle. Tell it not in Gath, for the elites will surely mock the revelation, but as for believers, shout if from the rooftops.

Chapter 9

Illation to Elation

As I began the process of putting together my thoughts for this book, friends would ask me, "What's your book going to be about, and what would be so compelling that you feel the need to get it in book form?" After I told them God revealed over three thousand years ago the same intermittent fasting eating patterns we see today, the overwhelming response was, "Really? You've got to be kidding! Tell me more!" Additionally, I was going to connect the eating patterns that were discovered in the 1800s with the same eating patterns that were studied extensively in the 2000s." Same message; two different millennia. I was going to show that *real science* absent cultural bias was going to prove God created us to thrive despite living in a fallen world.

In the 1800s, Dr. Dewey discovered the correct eating patterns but lacked the modern-day scientific evidence to substantiate his findings. In the 2000s, Dr. Mattson and other scientists, using the scientific method, were able to prove that the benefits of eating in very similar patterns as used in the 1800s were in fact true.

Both Dewey and Mattson proved time-restricted eating patterns were beneficial to those who chose to adopt them. One used decades of empirical evidence documenting the results of his patients, while the other used decades of scientific evidence that was catalogued and reviewed by fellow scientists in the laboratories of Johns Hopkins University. Where they differed was on the answer to the question as to *who* gets the credit. One gave credit to the divine, while the other gave credit to billions of years of atheistic, materialistic, Darwinian evolution. One gave credit to God, while the other gave credit to trillions of subsequent fortuitous accidents resulting in the evolution of organs that eventually came to be known as human bodies.

After reading both books, I was so intrigued by the results that I seriously considered giving it a try. I happened upon Exodus 16:21 during one of my morning devotions. At the same time, Dewey's and Mattson's findings were on the forefront of my mind since I had only recently discovered and read of their findings. I serendipitously found Dewey's book because Mattson had cited it in his work. While reading Exodus 16:21, it was as though a light came on. The fog was lifting, and I was seeing more clearly. I saw something I had never seen before. That's how the Holy Spirit works, you know, when you are studying God's Word; He often speaks to you in this way. We may dismiss it as an "aha" moment when it's actually the Holy Spirit revealing truths.

"So they gathered it every morning …" The children of Israel went out each day and gathered manna. I equated that with being active in the morning. "Every man according to his need. And when the sun became hot. It melted." I quickly went to my weather channel app and looked up the hourly heat in Jerusalem, and guess what? The hottest hour of the day is at 3:00 p.m. This is incredible; I am onto something:

- 3:00 p.m.—The day's supply of food melted.
- 7:00 a.m.—They would gather enough of the daily food for the entire family. (Let's say it took maybe an hour or two?)
- 8:00 a.m.—The seven-hour eating window begins.

What I discovered was that God had commanded the children of Israel to eat in a time-restricted eating pattern that is the same as a 17/7 intermittent fasting pattern just as Dr. Mattson espoused. Even if my assumptions were off by a couple of hours, they still would have been in an extended time of fasting. Their stomachs would have laid fallow, and they would have been in a ketogenic state, daily.

- 3:00 p.m.—The food melts.
- 3:00 a.m.—Their bodies flip the metabolic switch getting all the benefits that come along.

- 5:00 a.m.—Fourteen hours after their last meal, they gather the day's food having been in a ketogenic state for two hours.
- 6:00 a.m.—The nine-hour eating window begins, which means they had been in a ketogenic state for a full three hours.

Whether it was a 15/9, 16/8, or a 17/7 fast, they would still reap the benefits of being in a ketogenic state for either three, four, or five hours. That is a very similar percentage of time required of Israel to let the land lay fallow to allow it to rejuvenate itself. The question remains; were we and the rest of His creation created that way? Or were we just lucky to the trillionth degree?

I began to search the Bible to find out if it included other instances of this phenomena. The answer was yes. There are several examples. I was careful not to take the scriptures out of context to make scripture conform to my new breakthrough. Rather, I was ready and open to the fact that my theory might go up in smoke at the first sight of a contradiction. The thing is, I didn't find any. I soon discovered that the more the Holy Spirit revealed, the more I was convinced that all instances of eating in the Bible were in accordance with the pattern as outlined in Exodus 16:21.

When considering the scientific rule of Occam's razor (the simpler, the better), at least with the evidence I was able to gather, we see substantial proof that materialistic evolutionists are forced to contort their theory greatly to gain the support of the scientific community. In every account, they needed to explain away their theories, only to find out later the science would eventually catch up and authenticate what the Bible had been saying all along.

The one exception where I found God's people eating outside the Exodus 16:21 pattern was when God told Moses to get off His mountain because the children of Israel were behaving very badly. They were partying, eating, and drinking throughout the night as they worshiped their false gods and golden calf. Ecclesiastes tells us God was not at all happy when they weren't eating and drinking at the "proper time." (See Appendix 1.)

While some of the other stories in the Bible were not as directly put forth as the eating pattern of Exodus 16:21, one thing became very clear; every story we unwrapped in this book fits nicely within what I have come to believe is a preordained eating pattern, a gift from God to enable us to live healthier lives. A love story between God and His creation, if you will.

After considering all the evidence I was able to gather, I am compelled to come to the following inference. God created our finely tuned bodies in a finely tuned universe where we could dwell with Him forever. But because He gave us free will, we chose to disobey Him, which enabled sin to corrupt His perfect creation. Having known that we would do so, He had already created a means by which our bodies would heal themselves of many, but certainly not all, sickness and disease. All we need to do is follow the eating patterns as He demonstrated in His word: the Bible.

As for me, I've chosen to adopt the eating patterns as used by the children of Israel during their forty-year journey in the wilderness, and I couldn't be happier. At age fifty-seven, my physical well-being, increased energy, improved mental acuity, and overall health couldn't be better. This new eating pattern has changed my life for the better, and I plan on doing it for the rest of my life. I found in the Bible that God, the provider of every need, provided a way for our bodies to thrive in this fallen world. All we need to do is act on it.

Then God saw everything that He had made, and indeed [it was] very good. (Gen. 1:31 NKJV)

> Beloved, I pray that you may prosper in all things and be
> in health, just as your soul prospers. (3 John 1:2 NKJV)

> Rejoice in the Lord always. Again, I will say, rejoice! (Phil.
> 4:4 NKJV)

God wants His creation, you and I, to experience good health. Rejoice!

Appendices

1. Judgment occurred when food was eaten outside of the Exodus 16:21 eating pattern.

    Then they rose early on the next day, offered burnt offerings, and brought peace offerings; and the people sat down to eat and drink, and rose up to play. And the LORD said to Moses, "Go, get down! For your people whom you brought out of the land of Egypt have corrupted [themselves.] They have turned aside quickly out of the way which I commanded them. They have made themselves a molded calf, and worshiped it and sacrificed to it, and said, 'This [is] your god, O Israel, that brought you out of the land of Egypt!' And the LORD said to Moses, "I have seen this people, and indeed it [is] a stiff-necked people! Now therefore, let Me alone, that My wrath may burn hot against them and I may consume them. And I will make of you a great nation." (Ex. 32:6–10a NKJV)

    In Exodus 16:21, God taught the children of Israel to collect manna in the morning and eat during a window from 8:00 a.m. until 3:00 p.m. Here in Exodus 32, they were eating, drinking, and rising to play early in the morning. Rising to play are the Hebrew words *qum* and *sahaq*, which mean to arise and laugh, mock, or jest. They had "corrupted" themselves by eating, drinking, and carousing around their newly created golden calf. If it were not for Moses's pleading with God for their lives (v.11), God would have consumed them.

Woe to you, O land, when your king [is] a child, and
your princes feast in the morning! Blessed [are] you, O
land, when your king [is] the son of nobles, and your
princes feast at the proper time—For strength and not for
drunkenness! (Eccles. 10:16–17 NKJV)

Here in Ecclesiastes we read that God pronounced a curse on the
land because they worshiped idols while they feasted and drank in
the morning. He blessed the land when they worshiped God and
feasted at the proper time.

2. Introduction taken from *The True Science of Living* (Dewey 1893)
    by George F. Pentecost, DD.

The beloved apostle, writing to his well-beloved Gaius (3 John ii.),
whom he loves in the truth, greets him thus:

"Beloved, I wish above all things that thou mayest prosper
and be in health, even as thy soul prospereth."

Spiritual prosperity and health, which John takes for granted in
his salutation to his beloved Gaius, is certainly the highest blessing
attainable in this earth; but John prays that this great blessing may
be matched by another, namely the prosperity and health of the
body. It is with the sincerest desire that the readers of this book
may improve their health and increase their prosperity in body,
soul, and spirit that I have most willingly set my hand to write a
brief introduction to the pages of Dr. Dewey's book.

Bodily health is certainly desired by all men and women, especially
by those who have suffered from any loss of health or impairment
of physical strength. For the most part bodily health is desired
as a principal factor in our earthly enjoyment, and for the sake
of earthly gain and prosperity. But the Christian ought to desire
health of body for the higher reason that so he can serve God the
more efficiently. The body is the Lord's as well as the soul and
spirit. "He is the Saviour of the body also." "Know ye not that

your body is the temple of the Holy Ghost?" To defile the body with sin, or to voluntarily neglect the body in anywise as to cause it to suffer in health or strength, is an offence against our salvation and the honor of God. To deliberately undermine the health and strength of the body by persisting in an injurious, because false, way of living, is a sin of great enormity. Drunkenness or gluttony are offences against both body and soul which no self-respecting person, not to say Christian, ought for a moment to allow. Nevertheless, there are no doubt hundreds and thousands of good men and women who are guilty of both excess and bad methods in their eating and drinking that border upon these two disgusting and harmful sins.

The object of this book, as I understand it, is to put before the reader a "better way of living" than that which characterizes the great majority of people. It relates to the habit of eating and drinking, and sets forth from the point of view of sound physiology the relation of food to the human system, and so to disease and health.

If the author of this book is right in his premise and conclusion, he has set before the world a theory of living which ought to, and I believe will, revolutionize the habits of a multitude of right-thinking men and women. If he is right in supposing the coursing through our veins of pure, rich blood goes not only to preserve the health of the body and prolong life, but also that it makes for righteousness, both in clearing the mind and purifying the body of those humors which make fuel for unholy desires and unrighteous dispositions, then we must give attention to what he says. "Pure and rich blood (the life is in the blood) contributes to the moral, intellectual, and spiritual growth as well as to the bodily health." This proposition is almost self-evident and needs no argument. We should hail, then, with gladness, any discovery that will enable us to purify and enrich our blood.

Of the two principal matters recommended as the practical outcome of the theory of health developed in this book, the first is that fasting, or the abstinence from food until natural hunger calls for it, is the best way to bring about recovery from disease. Take away food from a sick man's stomach and you have begun, not to starve the sick man, but the disease. We have all of us heard that fevers are more difficult to subdue in large and full-habited people than in the "lean kind." I have often had my physician tell me that if ever typhoid or pneumonia got hold of me it would "'go hard with me," for the reason that there was so much material for the disease to feed upon. A conflagration is great or small in proportion to the quantity of easily-inflammable fuel the fire has to feed upon.

The second is that digestion is best promoted and food so assimilated as to afford the largest amount of nourishment and the greatest quantity of rich blood, by giving the stomach a long rest from all work during each twenty-four hours. That is to say that we shall be all the better by giving the stomach rest from the evening till the noon of the next day. In other words, Dr. Dewey recommends that we should give up our breakfasts, and by so doing we are certain to improve our health if we are well; prevent the incoming of disease; assist nature to recover from any unavoidable attack of sickness; strengthen the whole body, and thus build up the soul and the spirit which are so intimately connected with the body.

The only right I have to commend the book is the right which one man has who has tried the "better way of living" and has found that "it works well."

I am not personally acquainted with Dr. Dewey, the author of this book, but I have had the pleasure of some correspondence with him, and have experienced the benefit of greatly improved health by following out the simple rule of "right living" which he lays down in his pages. I am therefore quite ready to put my hand to an unconventional introduction, if by so doing I shall be enabled to induce any one to read these pages carefully; and, so far forth as the things therein contained applies to him, to follow the advice given faithfully.

When the blind man was asked by the Pharisees how Jesus opened his eyes, he related the fact of the process by which the miracle was wrought without attempting to explain the mystery of power underlying it. He answered and said, that "A man that is called Jesus made clay and anointed mine eyes and said unto me, go to the pool of Siloam and wash; and I went and washed, and I received sight."

And again, when the Pharisees cross-examined him, he repeated his simple testimony, "He put clay upon mine eyes and I washed and I do see." I am but a layman in the medical science and so do not pretend to discuss the subject professionally, but, as "a grateful patient," I am desirous of testifying to the benefits I have received from following Dr. Dewey's method of "right living."

This I know, that for forty years I have been a miserable victim of sick headache, induced by "a kind of indigestion," by "a torpid liver," by this and that, as I have been told by many physicians. I have tried every remedy and expedient that has in turn been recommended to me by physicians and friends. In many of them I have found temporary relief; but the cause of the trouble has ever remained, and the bilious sick headache, with its excruciating pain, would return and a total collapse of my power to work would supervene for from one to three or four days. I have tried dieting, that is not eating so heartily, not eating certain kinds of foods, not drinking coffee, etc. I have tried exercise of various kinds. I have tried preventive remedies, in the form of sodas of various kinds, antipyrins, antifebrins, pills, bromides of various kinds, etc. I have tried Turkish baths, and massage. All these things have given me more or less temporary relief, but I have always known that it was but temporary; that the real trouble was untouched. In addition to this bilious habit with its dread accompaniment of headaches, I have been steadily gaining in weight for twenty years past, until

I had reached the great weight, for a man of my height (5 feet 9 inches) of two hundred and fifty pounds. This has of course inconvenienced me, and brought on a certain shortness of breath upon the most moderate exertion either in walking or running, especially in running and going upstairs. I would not like to give the idea to any reader that I have been in any wise a sick man, for I have never, with the exception of the times when for a day or two I have been laid aside with sick headaches, been in bed a week in my life of fifty years, with any kind of sickness or disease according to the ordinary acceptation of these words. Indeed, I have been all my life a man of extraordinary health and strength, doing tremendous work in the line of my calling, preaching daily for months or years together to great crowds of people in every part of the world. At the same time, I have always been conscious of the fact that there was serious trouble behind this great store of health and strength, and especially has the steady accumulation of fat in my system been a source of anxiety as well as discomfort to me. The tendency to vertigo and a flushed face, and at times great lassitude which I could only overcome by great effort of will, has also caused me anxiety. I have been warned more than once by my doctors that I ought to be very careful not to make any great or violent exertion, as I was liable to suffer at any time from suffusion of blood upon the brain.

Well, some months ago, I chanced through a friend, whom I had known to be an invalid for years, and whom I then saw in seeming perfect health, to hear of Dr. Dewey and his method of "right living." I found that not only my friend, but every member of his family, including an invalid wife, a delicate daughter, two splendid young collegians, and a young boy of twelve had all given up eating their breakfasts; and that they were all greatly improved in health and strengthened mentally as well as physically. I was introduced by my friends to several other persons in his city who had adopted the "right living" method, and with one accord they all testified to the same great benefits experienced. I called on one or two business-men of my acquaintance who had adopted this method of living, and being men of my own type, they testified that they had, one and all, lost their tormenting sick headaches, lost a great deal of superficial fat and tissue, and were in every way greatly improved in health, in spirits, and in their capacity for work. I called upon an eminent physician whom I had known and who had on one or two occasions   prescribed for me. I asked him if he knew of Dr. Dewey's method of treatment and living. He said he did, and strongly recommended me to a adopt the anti-breakfast regime and confessed, sub-rosa, that he himself had adopted it, and was greatly the better for it. I learned of friends in my own calling who had suffered for years on Monday with fearful headaches because of physical and nervous exhaustion incident on their Sunday's work, who, having given up their breakfasts, had recovered entirely from the dreadful Monday prostrations and were enabled to do more and better work than ever before both in their studies and in their pulpits.

Taking the theory upon which this system of living is based into account (and even to my lay mind it seemed most reasonable), and the testimony which I personally received from both men and women, delicate and biliously strong, working-men, merchants, doctors and preachers, delicate ladies for years invalided and in a state of collapse, and some who had never been ill, but who were "an hundred percent better" for living without breakfast, I resolved to give up my breakfast. I pleaded at first that it might be my lunch instead, for I have all my life enjoyed my breakfast more than any other meal. But no! it was the breakfast that must go. So, on a certain fine Monday morning I bade farewell to the breakfast room. For a day or two I suffered slight headaches from what seemed to me was the want of food; but I soon found that they were just the dying pains of a bad habit. After a week had passed, I never thought of wanting breakfast; and though I was often present in the breakfast-rooms of friends with whom I was visiting, and every tempting luxury of the breakfast was spread before me, I did not desire food at all, feeling no suggestion of hunger.

Indeed now, after a few months the thought of breakfast never occurs to me. I am ready for my lunch (or breakfast if you please) at one o'clock, but I am never hungry before that hour. As for the results of this method of living I can only relate them as I have personally experienced them.

1. I have not had the first suggestion of a sick headache since I gave up my breakfast. From my earliest boyhood I do not remember ever having gone a whole month without being down with one of these attacks, and for thirty years, during the most active part of my life, I have suffered with them oftentimes, more or less every day for a month or six weeks at a time, and hardly ever a whole fortnight passed without an acute attack that has sent me to bed or at least left me to drag through the day with intense bodily suffering and mental discouragement.

2. I have gradually lost a large portion of my surplus fat, my weight having gone down some twenty pounds, and my size being reduced by several inches at the point where corpulence was the most prominent; and I am still losing weight and decreasing in size. The process of reduction is very gradual, but still is maintained from week to week.

3. I find that my skin is improving in texture, becoming softer, finer and more closely knit than heretofore. My complexion and eyes have cleared, and all fullness of the face and the tendency to flushness in the head has disappeared.

4. I experience no fullness and unpleasantness after eating as I so often did before. As a matter of fact, though I enjoy my meals (and I eat anything my appetite and taste call for) as never before, eating with zest, I do not think I eat as much as I used to do; but I am conscious of better digestion; my food does not lie so long in my stomach, and that useful organ seems to have gone out of the gas-producing business.

5. I am conscious of a lighter step and a more elastic spring in all my limbs. I can walk with quickness and for longer distances without consciousness of "that tired feeling" I used to experience. Indeed, a brisk walk now is a pleasure which I seek to gratify, whereas

before the prescribed walk for the sake of exercise was a horrible bore to me.

6. I go to my study and to my pulpit on an empty stomach without any sense of loss of strength mentally or physically; on the other hand, with freshness and vigor which is delightful. In this respect I am quite sure that I am in every way advantaged.

I may add, that, after seeing the manifest improvement that had taken place in my whole physical condition, my eldest daughter determined to follow in my footsteps, and she even went so far as to suggest to her little son (seven years old), that he also give up his breakfast. At first the wee chap said he wanted his breakfast and had a cry at the thought of being deprived of one of his natural and habitual rights. But his mother explained to him that she thought it would be a benefit to his health, and gave him a few simple reasons for the advice she had given him, and the little fellow pleasantly gave in to his mother. Nothing will induce him to eat his breakfast now till one o'clock, and both he and his mother are much better in health than before.

When I returned to England some months ago from America, my son, a lad of twenty, asked me why I did not eat my breakfast and I explained to him as best I could the theory of the "better living" system, beginning with the proposition that "restful sleep is not a hunger-causing process," and expounded also the advantage of a long rest for the stomach. I also pointed out to him that it is not the quantity of food which one eats that produces blood (good blood) and strength but the amount of nourishment which we get out of the food. After an hour's talk over the matter, without any recommendation or even suggestion on my part, and much less without thought that he would adopt this better method of living (for he was a great devotee to his breakfast) he said of his own accord: "Father, that seems a most sensible theory of living. I shall give up my breakfast at once."

Since then, he has eaten no breakfasts, and testifies to the fact that he feels a good fifty per cent better all the day through, and does his (office) work much easier and with a clearer head than before. He now playfully speaks of breakfast to his friends as "that vulgar habit."

One by one, of their own accord, every member of my family has given up their breakfast, and I think I can safely say that all are the better for it, though with one or two of them the sacrifice to the breakfast gods has been of so recent a date that I can only say they are the better on the principal of inductive philosophy.

My friends have, almost without an exception, noted and remarked upon the great improvement in my general health and appearance; and almost invariably said something like this: "How well you are looking." "Your holiday has done you a world of good." "Why, what have you been doing with yourself this summer? You are looking better than I ever saw you." "You must have been visiting the fountain of youth this summer. Tell me where it is and I will make a pilgrimage!" To these and similar remarks I have simply replied: "Oh, I have discovered the better way of living and been following it; and to that alone I attribute my general improvement in health and appearance." "What is it? Do tell me, for really, I am so dull and tired that life is sometimes a burden to me" (This remark is literally quoted.). "Well, it is very simple. Just give up eating your breakfast."

"What, give up my breakfast!" "Why I would rather give up any other meal in the day. Besides I could never do my work without my breakfast." "I should faint before ten o'clock." "It is quite true that I eat very little breakfast, but I am sure I could never get through the morning without it." "Oh, that may do very well for a great healthy man like you, but I could never manage it."

These are specimen answers, quoted literally; to which I have replied invariably by a brief statement of the anti-breakfast theory and then expounded; beginning with "Restful sleep is not a hunger causing process," and going on to suggest that the breakfast they eat cannot furnish strength for them to do their morning work upon, as in no case does food give strength until it is converted into blood. That we all do our work today largely if not entirely on the blood extracted from the food of yesterday. Then I have questioned them as to their habits and state of health, and in nine cases out of ten I have found that these friends of mine, the more healthy ones as well as the delicate ones, all suffer in some degree from some one of the many forms of indigestion. Headaches, palpitation, fullness of habit, neuralgia, accumulation of gas in the stomach, pimples on the face, or some other form of eczema arising from and due to poor blood. These conversations have always awakened interest, and even the most skeptical have again returned to the discussion of the matter, as though the very mention of the matter had produced conviction.

In at least a score of cases my friends have adopted the "right-living" method, and all testify to their great delight in it. In one or two cases where dyspepsia has been a veritable fiend, and health and strength almost gone, with depression of mind and even decay of will, the improvement has been most marked, and these friends are on the high-road to health again. I could fill pages of interesting details coming under my own observation and resulting from the adoption of the rule, on the strength of my simple expositions, which would be surprising.

I am often asked if it is possible that I preach on Sundays, that is in the morning, without any food, as though that were a feat almost incredible. To which I am able not only to say, "Yes, of course," but more than that, "I go to my pulpit fresher in body and mind, and come out of it fresher after the sermon, than I ever did in the old breakfast-eating days."

I have come to the conclusion that the blood cannot take care of the brain and the stomach at the same time, and if a man has a breakfast to digest and a sermon to preach during the same period of time, either the breakfast or the sermon will have to suffer, and most likely both of them do. So convinced am I of this fact that I am almost prepared to believe that preachers would do better work and be stronger in body if, as a rule, they took no food at all on Sundays, but only drank what they cared for of water. A twenty-four-hour fast from all food once a week would not only do no harm, but would give the stomach such a rest as would enable all the other bodily functions to clear the body of unhealthy remainders. God has ordained a seventh-day fast from exhausting and secular labor. Of old He ordained a fast once in seven years for the land that it might recover and recoup itself from too constant labor of production. We know that all ship owners and other users of machinery require their engines and boilers to have an occasional rest. Two pairs of boots will wear longer, if the use of them is alternated, than three pairs worn steadily, one pair after the other till each is worn out. Why then is it unreasonable to suppose that it is a good thing to give the stomach, that most delicate and important of all our organs, as long a rest each day as possible, and occasionally a much longer rest! Some of my friends have charged me with having fallen into the hands of a "quack," and have thrown this at me: "If this anti-breakfast theory for people who are not invalids, and the ' starvation theory' for sick people were true, do you suppose that it would have been left for an obscure country doctor in America to have discovered it? Have any of the great medical authorities, such as Sir A. B. and C. D. and Q. X., recommended?" In a word, "Have any of the rulers believed on him?" I do not pretend to argue the matter technically as I am not a technically educated physician. Therefore, my testimony is that of a layman. As such I give it for what it is worth. I cannot help, however, thinking again of the case of the blind man who was questioned by the Pharisees. They had a theory that Jesus must be a bad man and a sinner because He healed on the Sabbath day, which to them was the most sacred thing they possessed, more sacred than God Himself. The man that was born blind and yet was restored to sight replied very wisely, as a layman: "Whether he be a sinner or not, I know not; one thing I know, that whereas I was blind, now I see."

It is even so in such a case as this. Here is a man with a theory for "better living," which he is prepared to defend on scientific principles, and to demonstrate by actual experimental evidence. Here is a theory of "better living" which I and scores of others have tried, so simple, so full of common sense, and withal one which we have demonstrated by a simple experimental test. The theory may not be endorsed by the medical profession, nor widely acted upon by practitioners, but since "it works well" with all sorts and conditions of patients, we are bound to say again with the blind man, modifying his words a little, "Why, here is a marvelous thing, that ye know not whence this 'better way of living'" comes from, yet it giveth better health and enables nature to cure innumerable diseases that have in other patients proved fatal, simply by letting her take her own course and not worrying her by over-feeding a diseased stomach and lashing it as a cabby does his tired and jaded horse.

For the benefit of my fellow-ministers, into whose hands this book I hope will fall, I pass Dr. Dewey's Prescription to me, on to them."

Always go into your study, your pulpit, and your bed with an empty stomach. Follow this rule as nearly as you can, and I will guarantee the largest measure of health and strength that is possible in your case. "In any case I most seriously and heartily recommend that one and all of the readers of this book give up eating breakfast, and they will know in themselves in less than two months whether the doctrine be based on sound principles or whether it be the vagary of a quack. "The proof of the pudding is in the eating." It certainly will do no one any harm to leave off the breakfast for three months and it is equally almost certain that before that time has elapsed any one so doing will need no further argument.

—George F. Pentecost
London England
November 9, 1894

References

Anstey, Martin. 1973. *Chronology of the Old Testament.* Grand Rapids, MI: Kregel Publications.

Clarey, Dr. Timothy. 2015. *Dinosaurs: Marvels of God's Design.* Arizona: Master Books.

Clarey, Dr. Timothy. 2020. *Carved in Stone: Geological Evidence of the Worldwide Flood.* Dallas: Institute for Creation Research.

Collins, Francis S. 2006. *The Language of God.* New York: Free Press.

DeHaan, M. R. 1970. *The Romance of Redemption: The Love Story of Ruth and Boaz.* Grand

Rapids, MI: Zondervan.

Dewey, Edward Hooker. 1894. *The True Science of Living: The New Gospel of Health, Practical and Physiological; Story of an Evolution of Natural Law in the Cure of Disease, for Physicians and Laymen.* London: Henry Bill.

Foreman, Matt, and Doug Van Dorn. 2020. *The Angel of the Lord.* Dacono, Colorado: Waters of Creation.

Fruchtenbaum, Arnold G. 2021. *Ariel's Bible Commentary: The Book of Genesis.* San Antonio: TX: Ariel Ministries.

Mattson, Mark P. 2022. *The Intermittent Fasting Revolution: The Science of Optimizing Health and Enhancing Performance.* Cambridge, MA: MIT Press.

Metaxas, Eric. 2021. *Is Atheism Dead?* Washington, DC: Salem Books.

Tsarfati, Amir. 2022. *Revealing Revelation: How God's Plan for the Future Can Change Your Life Now.* Eugene, OR: Harvest House.

Whiston, William A. M. 1737. *The Genuine Works of Flavius Josephus the Jewish Historian.* London.

1. 6:00 a.m.: Coffee and devotion.

   No cream or sugar in your morning drink if you can (no energy intake including juices of any kind). Zero calorie artificial sweetener is OK. If you are a type 1 diabetic, do not follow this pattern. Do only as recommended by your doctor. Type 2 is a different story. Go for it! It will make you feel better.

2. 7:00 a.m.: Flip the switch.

   Your body has now "flipped the metabolic switch" and is creating and burning ketones rather than the 400 to 500 calories of glucose that was stored in your liver. You are in a ketogenic state because your last energy intake was twelve hours ago. This is a great place to be.

   Moderate exercise if you can. If you exercise in a ketogenic state, the results will yield exponential health benefits.

3. 7:30 a.m.: Start your energy-filled day.

   If you have not had any caloric intake, you are still in a ketogenic state. Begin your day with a water regimen to keep you satisfied until you break your fast. Zero calorie soft drinks are OK on occasion. If you must have some cream in your coffee early in the morning, no worries. You can easily burn those calories and get back in your optimal state.

   When you feel that stomach growling, rejoice! Use that feeling to remind you of all the miracles that are taking place inside your body at this very moment. You will learn to love it.

4. 10:00 a.m.-noon: Break your fast—if you want to.

   Begin enjoying your seven- to nine-hour eating window. It's marvelous.

5. 7:00 p.m.: Finish your last meal of the day.

No late-night snacks.

Starting out you may want to use a 15–9 eating pattern. After your last meal of the day, break your fast fifteen hours after energy intake, where you will enjoy a nine-hour eating window. By doing this pattern, you will still have "flipped the switch" for three hours each day getting all the benefits that come. If and when you're able, you can try working your way up to a 17–7 eating pattern. This pattern will result in your body benefitting from being in a ketogenic state for five to seven hours each day. If you would like to have breakfast in the church café on Sunday morning, please do. Fellowship is too important. Anyhow, God didn't melt the manna the night before the Sabbath, so it's not out of the realm of possibility that they enjoyed quail eggs and manna waffles the very next morning. Besides, you still benefited by getting your body in its optimal state for six full days. You are going to feel great.

* Intermittent fasting could have significant health benefits for those suffering with type 2 diabetes. If you have been diagnosed with type 1 diabetes, please consult with your physician before adopting time-restricted eating patterns.